Mad Skills
Exercise Encyclopedia

Ben Musholt

First published in 2013 by BPM Rx, Inc.

ISBN 13: 978-1492139409
ISBN 10: 1492139408

Cover design by Miguel Aldana
www.SlowFastGo.com
Illustrations and layout by Diego G. Diaz
www.diegogdiaz.com

BPM Rx and Strength Mob are registered trademarks of BPM Rx, Inc.

DISCLAIMER:
This book is for educational purposes only. The publisher and author are not responsible in any manner whatsoever for any adverse effects arising directly or indirectly as a result of the information contained within the book. The exercises and the movements covered in this book can be dangerous to yourself and your training partners if not performed with correct form, safety, and caution. Consultation with a qualified fitness professional is recommended prior to beginning any training. Likewise, you are advised to consult with physician before starting this or any other exercise program.

Your health and safety are of paramount importance. Be smart: Train with caution, and use appropriate exercise progressions.

For my beautiful wife, Lorraine.

Your support and encouragement are the reason that this book is a reality. I'm blessed to be your partner.

Special thanks to all of the amazing models that have lent their image to this exercise encyclopedia:

Chris Bibro, Johanna Bibro, Jessica Chang, Aaron Cooper, Laney Coyne, Lorraine Escribano, Casey Frieder, Jamie Minkus, Sara Mohkami, Laura Musholt, Aaron Ogden, Ryan Pennington, Senna Pinney, Jake Reid, Aaron Saari, Alexis Saari, Gloria Trujillo, Ramman Turner, Jimmy Udall, Xi Xia

Table of Contents

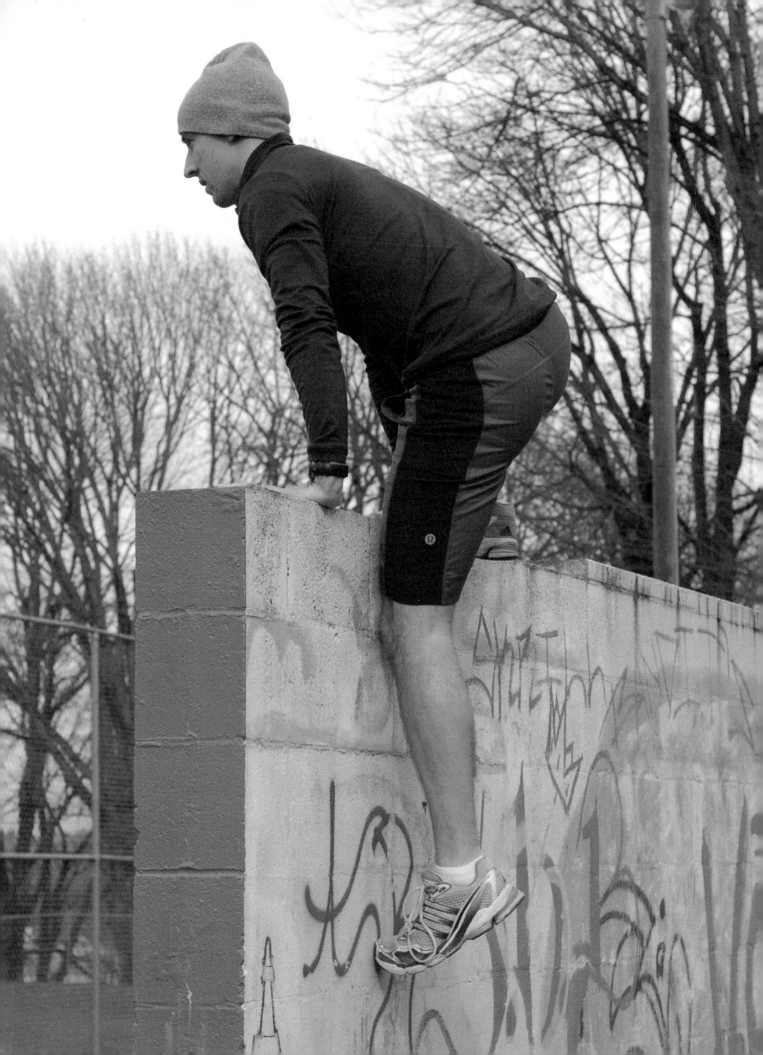

Preface
Movement is my mistress.

Our relationship began when I was nine months old, rolling my infant walker down the sloped floor of my parents' apartment. By five years old, my alluring partner in motion had me climbing doorframes and hallways. Years six through twelve we made the pact to master the martial arts. As a high schooler, she helped me claim the Wisconsin state freshman gymnastics title for parallel bars. In my later teenage years, she had me throwing double twisting somersaults from the diving board. And, at college in New Mexico, she enticed me to launch my snowboard-strapped body from big cliffs.

No matter what hardship I've suffered, she has always been at my side, ready to console with a solid trail run or some old-school calisthenics. In our more intimate moments, we've explored yoga, skateboarding, surfing, and capoeira. Her drug is irresistible, but don't get me wrong — we've had our bad moments. Two shoulder surgeries and a bone sticking out of my knee are some of the worst injuries I suffered from our tangles.

I'm thirty-five years old now, happily married with a respectable career as a physical therapist, but my mistress and I still get together now and then. Sometimes we'll catch up at the local bouldering gym or escape together for a bit of impromptu acrobatics. Not that my wife doesn't notice. She does. But thankfully she turns a blind eye to my fooling around. What can I say? I guess she knows some relationships are impossible to untangle.

Mad Skills is not a treatise about the love of movement — I would have to write that at in some other more creative context. It is my professional attempt to give you the skills to be fit enough to pursue your love of movement, at whatever pace or vigor that you choose.

The stronger and more flexible you are, the better you can move. Period.

What you and movement choose to do in your private time . . . that's none of my business.

Ben Musholt
Portland, OR
September, 2013

"The hundreds of exercises that will be introduced in Mad Skills are meant to enhance your baseline physical fitness."

Introduction

This is not the fitness book you need if you've got to lose weight for a wedding or get your body beach-ready for spring break. Within these pages you won't find any advice on fat loss. Nor are there any secret tricks for sculpting your six-pack. I won't tell you how to run a faster half-marathon either. Same thing goes for diet plans.

You won't find any of that in here.

There are plenty of other books that cover those topics and I'm just not excited about that stuff anyhow.

On the other hand, if you're a seasoned athlete and are looking for a kick in the pants—something to take your skills to the next level—look no further. What you are holding is an exercise encyclopedia for the new fitness revolution. Within its covers there are over 700 killer body weight and free weight movements for building strength and mobility.

Whether you ski off-piste, train MMA, or compete in adventure races, this is the reference tool you need on your bookshelf. Its aim is to open your eyes to hundreds of different ways to move, strengthen, and enhance your body's ability to function in both daily life and on the playing field.

The broader array of movement skills that you train, the better athlete you will be.

This statement sums up the entire reason for the existence of this book.

From barbell lifts, kettlebell movements, gymnastics skills, and even basic calisthenics, *Mad Skills* will broaden your strength-training repertoire. And, with dozens of unique stretches and yoga postures, you should come away with a few new ideas for how to keep your body limber and ready for whatever you throw its way.

There is no need to read this book cover to cover. It's meant to be flipped through, highlighted, and dog-eared as you jump between chapters, looking for new movements to add to your workouts. If you're a fitness professional or athletic coach, keep it handy for when you want to challenge someone with a fresh exercise. Heck, go ahead and use it for coffee table decoration—the illustrations are cool enough that your guests should be impressed for years to come.

Why You Won't Find Recommendations for Weights, Reps, Sets, Et Cetera

Although the last chapter of the book will suggest a way to tie all of the exercises together into different workouts, this book will not prescribe a specific way to bulk up, prepare for competition, or improve a sport-specific skill set. You won't find recommendations for kilograms to lift, number of sets to perform, or how many specific reps to complete. Those types of recommendations must be tailored to each individual, taking into account one's goals and starting point. *However, this book should be considered a supplement to any sport-specific conditioning you are already doing.*

The goal of *Mad Skills* is to introduce a huge variety of unique workout movements. That's it. If you're looking for advice on enhancing performance within a given athletic activity, your best bet is to meet with a coach in that field. Based on your specific goals, an expert can craft a workout routine that helps you build, taper, and achieve your desired outcome.

The hundreds of exercises that will be introduced in *Mad Skills* are meant to enhance your baseline physical fitness. By rotating through a plentiful set of complex and varied exercise skills, you sharpen your nervous system, strengthen your joints, and build muscle memory for a large movement repertoire.

Physical performance in any athletic situation is determined by how much preparation you've done prior to the event, coupled with your natural talent. By utilizing a numerous variety of movement skills in your training, you give yourself an advantage over someone with a smaller movement repertoire. Whether it's tug-of-war, cyclo-cross, or flag football, the greater variety of training you've done, the better your likelihood of succeeding in the unique challenges of the activity.

Fitness, Not (P)Rehab

I'm a physical therapist by trade, so prescribing movements to help people prevent or recover from injury is near and dear to my heart. But, for better or for worse, that is not the purpose of this book. The exercise selection used to help people rehabilitate from an injury is quite diverse, and includes movement techniques that go beyond the scope of this encyclopedia.

You're not going to find any movements in these pages that use resistance bands or focus on joint stabilization. I love those skills. They're great, but they just don't have a place in this particular collection. It would take at least another two hundred pages to describe the variety of movements that rehab professionals use to help the injured.

Start Where You Are

You'll find that the majority of the skills in the next chapters can be done at home or in your garage with a limited set of tools. I've been growing my supply of weights and exercise equipment over a number of years, which has prevented any large up-front costs associated with my fitness pursuits. Perhaps you've got your own collection of dumbbells tucked away somewhere?

If the idea of going out and buying a ton of workout equipment is daunting, don't worry—often one piece of equipment can be used for multiple purposes. Also, consider spreading costs out among your workout buddies. If everyone chips in with the equipment they have, one person's garage could be outfitted as an awesome resource for the community.

Here is a list of some of the equipment you'll see used in *Mad Skills:*

- Dumbbells
- Barbells + weight plates
- Kettlebells
- Pull-up bar
- Gymnastics rings
- Parallette bars
- Medicine balls

- Yoga mat
- Weight bench
- Sandbag
- Stability ball
  (also known as a Physioball or a Swiss ball)
- Plyometric box (referred to as a plyo box)

Individuals who have followed strength and conditioning trends over the last few years might be shocked to see that missing from this list are tires (to flip), sledge hammers (to swing), or heavy ropes (to shake). Those omissions were intentional. All of the exercises you'll find in *Mad Skills* were selected so that someone with limited space or resources could improve his or her fitness without having access to a large, well-stocked gym.

You should be able to substitute many of the pieces of equipment in the list for an alternate if you don't have the funds or the storage to purchase and house everything. A stability ball can often be swapped for a weight bench. Likewise, dumbbells can replace kettlebells when needed. In a pinch, your neighborhood park can even be a great resource with different exercise tools, like benches, pull-up bars, and jungle gym features.

Get After It!

The aim of this book is to provide you with an illustrated resource for an abundance of strength and conditioning ideas. Hopefully, it will become your trusted companion for when you need some inspiration for a new workout. Jump right in, try the moves out, and discover how varying your exercise routine pays dividends on your athletic performance. Whether you throw back flips for fun, shred the slopes, or play intramural soccer, I hope that the moves in *Mad Skills* improve your skill level in whatever sport brings you joy.

Chapter 1

"Pull on the tracksuit and slip on your sweatbands. It's time to get down to action."

Fire It Up!

Pull on the tracksuit and slip on your sweatbands. It's time to get down to action. Before jumping into any physical activity it's critical to perform a series of motions to prepare your joints and muscles for the upcoming strain. How long and how intense you perform a "warm-up" is dependent on what you plan to be doing. If you're going to be training aerials on the freestyle ski slope, you'd better be sure to wake up your nervous system and get your limbs ready to absorb major shock. Just taking off for a simple trail run? Starting off slow for the first few minutes might be all you need.

For the context of designing a workout to build strength and general physical preparedness, a warm-up should entail 5 to 10 minutes of rhythmic body-weight movement. The rhythmic element is important so that you raise your internal temperature. An elevated body temperature lets your muscles function more effectively.

The restriction to body weight is meant to prevent you from exhausting your energy supplies prior to beginning the larger part of your workout routine. Ideally, in a thorough warm-up, you should move your arms, legs, trunk, and neck in a way to prepare them for the exercises of the next portion of your workout.

A good target is to move enough that you've broken a slight sweat, prior to moving onto other workout activities.

The 50+ movements in this section have been divided into those that are performed while standing, versus those that you do when on the ground. Many of the movements could be combined to create a solid body weight circuit without even jumping into the next chapters. However, the purpose here is to give you some ideas of simple movements in preparation for the heavier, fun stuff.

It is important to note that there really isn't a single warm-up skill that utilizes 100% of each joint. To be effective, you usually need to pair an upper body warm-up skill, with a lower body one. Sometimes, even 3 to 4 movements will be needed to constitute a thorough warm-up. Be creative!

Leg Swing

- Swing one leg forward and backward.
- Take the leg through as much range of motion as possible, building up to a larger and larger arc of motion.
- Hold a wall or chair for balance, as needed.
- Do both sides.

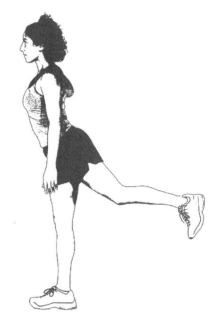

Lateral Leg Swing

- Place your hands on a wall at chest height, for support.
- Swing one leg side to side in front of your body.
- Work a progressively larger arc of motion, for a good dynamic stretch of the inner and outer leg.

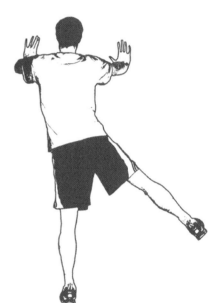

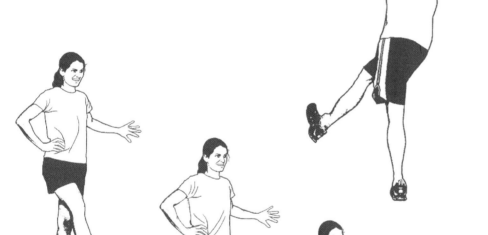

Hip Circles

- Raise a leg out to the side and move it around in clockwise and counter-clockwise directions.
- Work it through a small and large range of motion.
- Hold a wall or chair for balance.

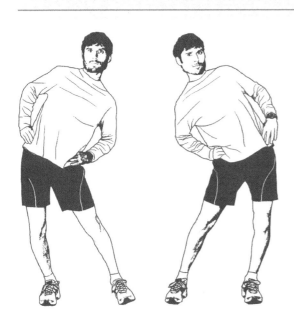

Pelvis Circles

- Stand with feet shoulder-width apart.
- Circle your trunk and pelvis around in large circles.
- Make sure to go in both directions, and work as much motion as possible.

Trunk Circles

- Stand with feet slightly wider that shoulder-width apart.
- Raise arms above your head.
- Move your trunk in a large circle, reaching backward then dropping forward to sweep the ground.
- Keep your abdominal muscles tight to protect your low back.

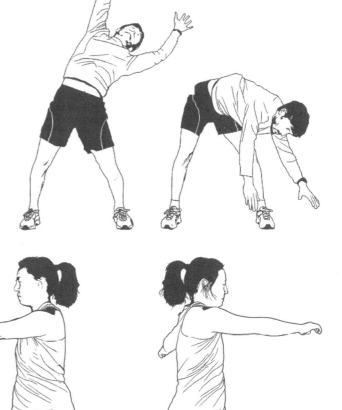

Trunk Twist

- Stand with your feet shoulder-width apart and your arms spread wide, held at chest level.
- Rotate your trunk to one side and reach your opposite hand across your body for an extra twist.
- Repeat on the other side and continue back and forth, engaging your trunk muscles.

Bent Over Twist

- Spread your feet double-shoulder width apart and bend forward at your waist.
- Reach one hand to the floor, twist your trunk to the side, and raise your other hand to the ceiling.
- Twist to the other side and switch hand positions.
- Repeat back and forth, engaging your trunk muscles.

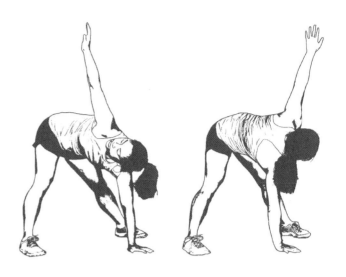

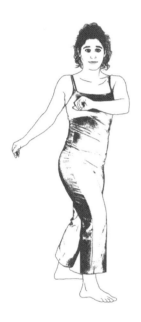
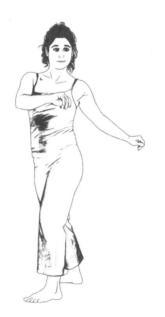

Twisting Jumps

- Jump up and down while twisting your lower body from one side to the other.
- Swing your arms in the opposite direction of your lower body.

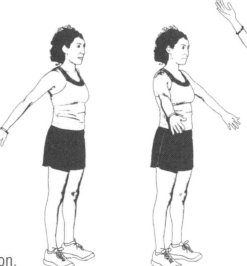

Arm Circles

- Rotate both shoulders in a wide circles.
- Move in as big a loop as possible.
- Switch directions every few rotationsepetitions.
- Variation: Do just one arm and allow more trunk rotation.

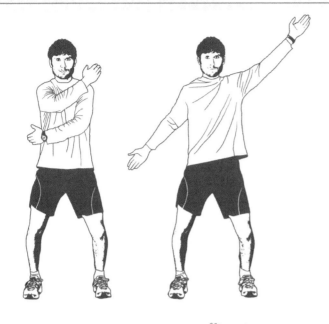

Diagonal Shoulder Swings

- Start with your arms crossed in front of your body.
- Spread your arms apart, along a diagonal, and then return your arms to the original position.
- Let your shoulder blades glide forward and backward along your ribcage for extra movement.
- Work your full range of motion, and then switch sides.

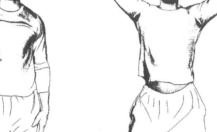

Jumping Jacks

- Start with your hands at your side and feet together.
- Jump upward, while spreading your hands and feet.
- Touch hands together, while your feet strike the ground.
- Jump back to the starting position.
- Repeat for time or repetitions.

Split Jacks

- Start by standing with one leg in front of the other.
- Jump up and explosively switch legs, dropping down into a slight lunge.
- Move your arms at the same time as the your legs.
- Your arms should move opposite of your legs.

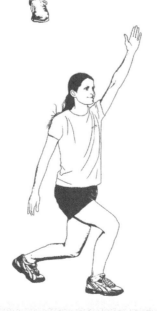
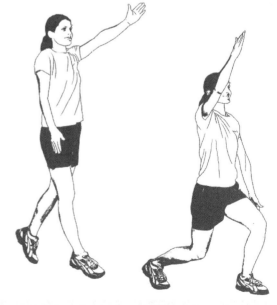

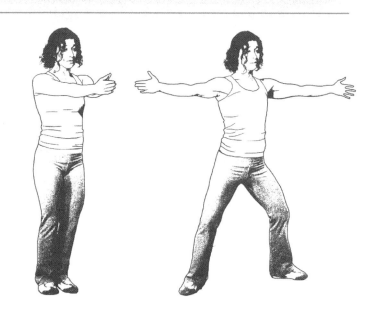

Commando Jacks

- Start by standing with your feet together and your hands extended in front of your chest, with your palms touching.
- Jump up and spread your arms and legs apart.
- Hop back to the beginning position, clapping your feet and hands together

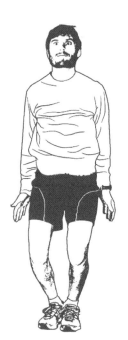

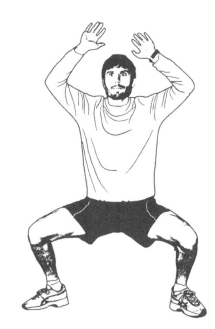

Sumo Squat Jumping Jacks

- Similar to regular jumping jacks, but you drop lower.
- Your legs should be spread open into a "sumo squat" position, with your toes pointed out slightly.

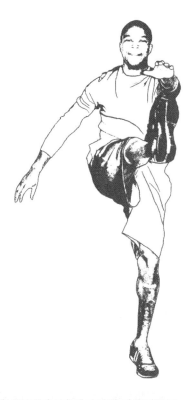

Squat Kick

- Start in a medium depth squat.
- Your feet should be positioned hip distance apart or wider.
- As you stand up, swing one leg up to touch your opposite hand.
- Alternate sides on each repetition.

Toe Taps

- Use a medicine ball, stack of weights,   dumbbell, or a stair as a target.
- Hop up and down — alternating which foot touches the target.
- Keep your hands behind your head for extra effort.

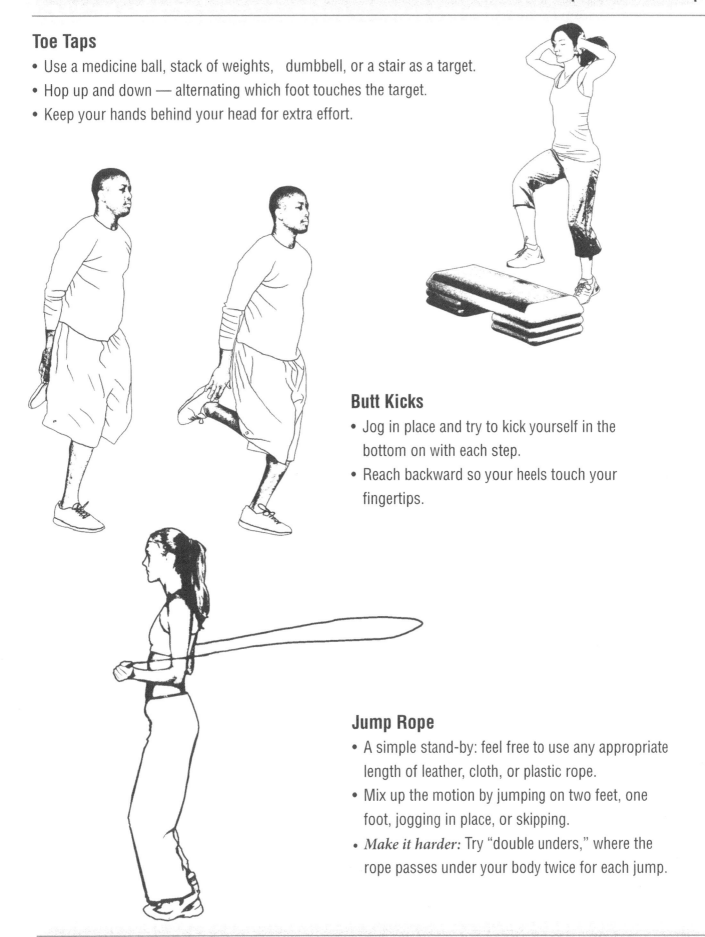

Butt Kicks

- Jog in place and try to kick yourself in the bottom on with each step.
- Reach backward so your heels touch your fingertips.

Jump Rope

- A simple stand-by: feel free to use any appropriate length of leather, cloth, or plastic rope.
- Mix up the motion by jumping on two feet, one foot, jogging in place, or skipping.
- *Make it harder*: Try "double unders," where the rope passes under your body twice for each jump.

Run

- Get your heart rate up with some basic jogging.
- Start slow, and then build to running speed.
- Pump your arms for whole-body involvement.

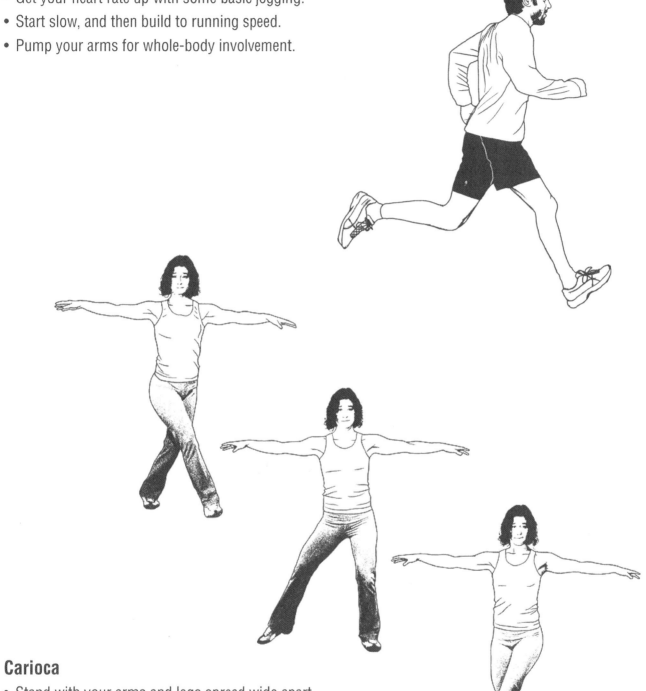

Carioca

- Stand with your arms and legs spread wide apart.
- Step one leg across the front of the other leg.
- Then, step your back leg out the side, so that you begin to move sideways.
- Step your first leg behind the second, continuing your sideways motion.
- This movement is also known as the "Grapevine."

Shadow Box

- Imitate a boxer's pose by moving around throwing air punches.
- Think about your footwork, moving through small semi-circles.
- Switch up your jabs with hooks and uppercuts.
- *Variation:* Add kicks, plus elbow and knee strikes.

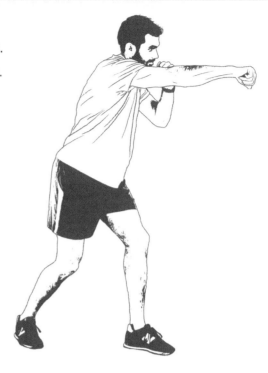

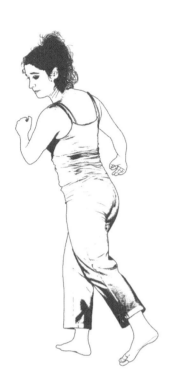

Backward Run

- Look over one shoulder and begin to jog backwards.
- Emphasize strong hip extension, and reach for the ground with your toes.
- Run in a circle for a few laps, and then switch directions to work both sides equally.

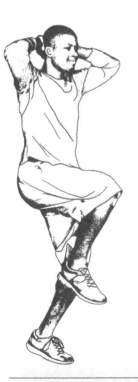
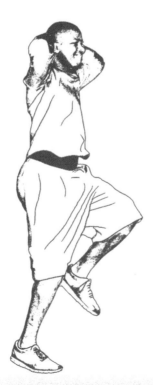

High Stepping

- Interlace your fingers behind your head.
- Hop back and forth, marching your knees high.
- Strive to get your knees to at least pelvis level.
- You can do this in place or while moving forward.

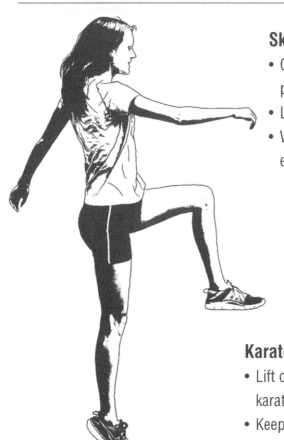

Skip

- Channel your inner child and propel yourself forward and upward, pushing forcefully off one leg.
- Lift your other leg high while pumping your arms.
- Work on spanning a long distance, while also going for height on each step.

Karate Skip

- Lift one leg to the "ready" position of a karate stance.
- Keep your fists by your face.
- Skip forward on your back leg, hopping along on one leg.
- *Make it harder*: Add a kicking motion with the elevated leg.

Lunge Kick

- Start in a medium depth lunge with both hands up, on guard.
- Push off the back leg and swing it forward to perform a kick.
- Drive your hips forward in a thrusting movement.
- Return the kicking leg to the backward position.

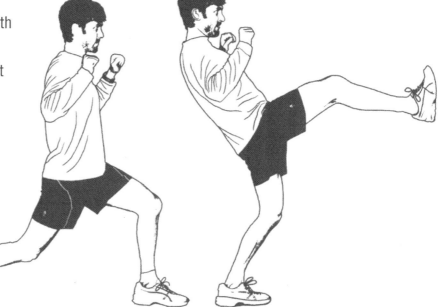

Twisting Lunge

- Stand with your feet together and your arms held in front of your chest, with your palms touching.
- Take a large step forward into a lunge.
- Rotate your trunk and arms over the side of the front leg.
- Return to the starting position.
- Repeat on the other side.
- *Variation:* Walk forward as you perform the twisting lunges.

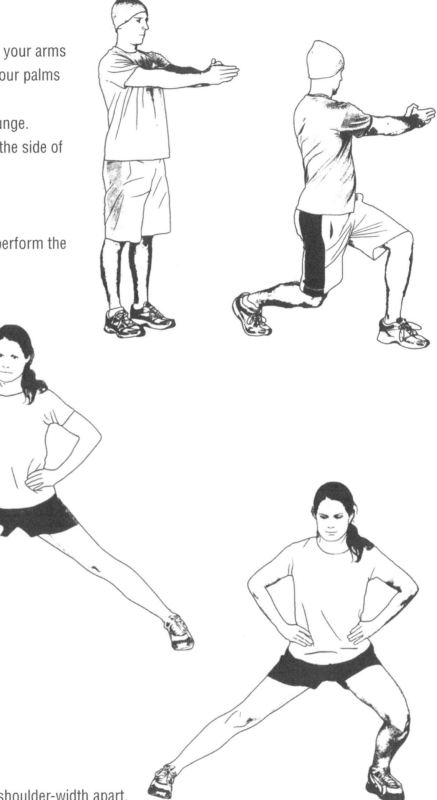

Side to Side Lunges

- Spread your feet at least double shoulder-width apart.
- Move to one side while bending a knee to drop into a side lunge.
- Push back to the middle and lunge to the opposite side.
- Watch your knee alignment so the leg doesn't drop inward.

Speed Skater Jumps

- Imitate the motion of a speed skater by jumping side to side.
- Land in a slight crouch with the opposite arm swinging across your body.
- Keep tight so that you don't have too much vertical chest movement.
- Stay low and monitor your knee alignment.

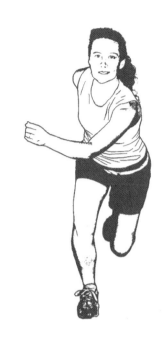 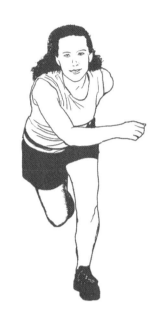

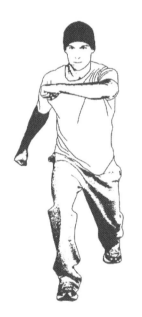 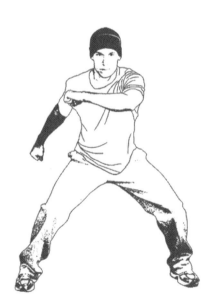 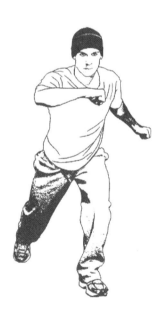

Ginga

- Start in a lunge position with the arm on the same side as your back leg held in front of your body.
- Step out to the side, into a wide-legged stance.
- Retract the leg that had been forward, place it on the ground behind you, and switch arm positions.
- Your steps should trace the points of an isosceles triangle.

Marching Knee Tucks

- March in place while pulling your knees to your chest.
- Alternate back and forth.
- Stretch your knees and hips by holding each movement for a few seconds.

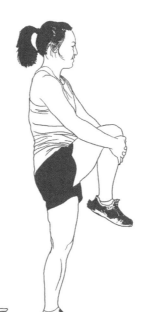
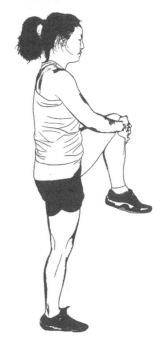

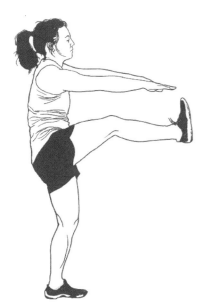
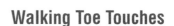

Walking Toe Touches

- Walk forward while swinging your feet up to touch your hands.
- Don't let your back round too much.
- Try to keep your knees straight to stretch your hamstrings.

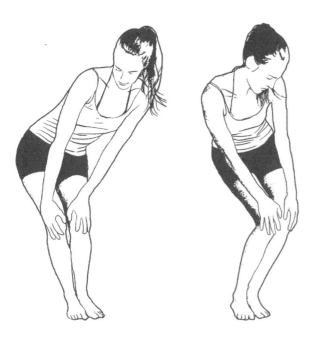

Knee Circles

- Stand with your feet together and your knees slightly flexed.
- Bend forward and place your hands on your lower thighs.
- Keep your knees together and rotate them in progressively wider circles.
- Rotate in both directions, gently preparing your knee cartilage and ligaments for greater activity.
- *Variation:* Instead of moving in circles, try to spread your knees apart and back together in an outward/inward motion.

Knee Bends

- Stand with your feet together and your hands placed on your lower thighs.
- Bend your knees, lowering your bottom toward your heels.
- Allow your heels to come off the floor and let your legs spread for greater depth.
- Return to standing and then lower down again, trying to go deeper on each squat.

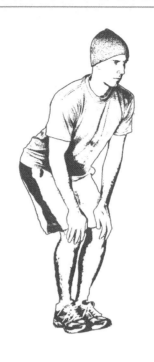
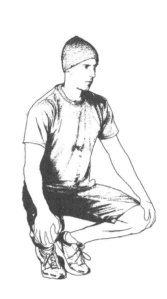

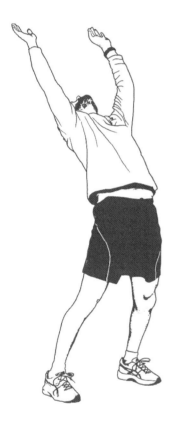

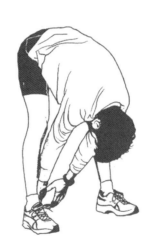

Reaching Backbend

- Stand with legs hip-width apart.
- Tighten your abdominal muscles to protect your low back.
- Reach your arms overhead while extending your trunk into a backbend.
- Collapse forward, reaching your hands between your legs.
- *Variation:* Bounce downward a few beats, touching different points on the ground.

Duckwalk

- Squat low with your hands above your head.
- Step forward with one leg, while keeping your bottom down.
- Keep your knees as low as possible, while stepping through on each step.

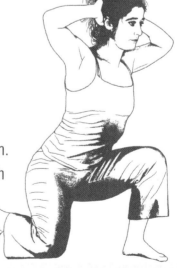

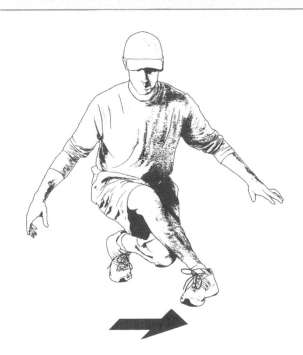

Crouched Side Step

- Crouch down in a low squat.
- Step one foot across the other, initiating movement to one side.
- Keep your bottom low in a crouched position as you step laterally.
- Avoid injury by being conscious of your knee alignment.

Frog Hop

- Balance on your forefeet in a low squat.
- Hop forward while trying to land as softly as possible.
- Keep your bottom/thigh angle below 90 degrees.
- *Variation:* Vary your bounces along diagonals.

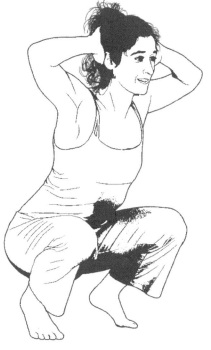

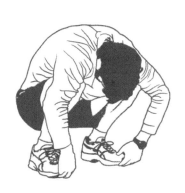

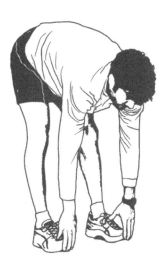

Squat to Stand

- Begin in a low squat position with your fingertips by your toes.
- Let your spine curve, allowing your chin to drop to your chest
- Lift your bottom into the air to elongate your hamstrings.

Knee to Face

- Begin in a high 3-point plank position with one leg elevated behind you.
- Bring the elevated knee to your face while rounding your back.
- Push hard through your arms and extend backward to the starting position.

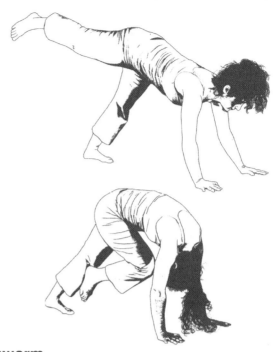

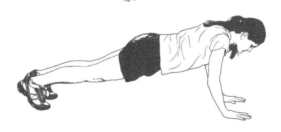

Inchworm

- Start in a forward bend.
- Walk your hands outward while bringing your pelvis to horizontal.
- Finish in a plank position, staying tight through your trunk and hips.
- Walk your feet up to your hands so that you progress forward along the floor.

Forearm Crawl

- Drop to your forearms in a low plank position.
- Crawl forward, trying to keep your trunk and hips as low as possible.
- Pretend you are crawling through a narrow tunnel.

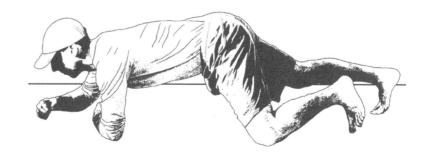

Alligator Crawl

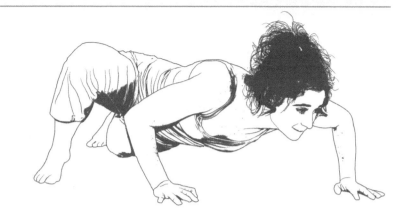

- Similar to the forearm crawl, but with your palms on the ground.
- Keep your torso and pelvis low as you crawl one arm/leg forward at a time.
- Imagine you are wiggling below strings of barbed wire, as in a military boot camp.

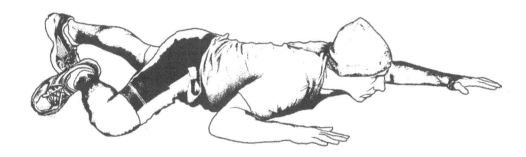

Belly Crawl

- Begin on the floor with your belly touching the ground and your limbs spread apart ready to move.
- Move your opposite arm and leg forward along the ground.
- Continue creeping forward while trying to keep your pelvis down to the ground.
- Think of it as a super low "Commando Crawl" to help you get through a narrow space.

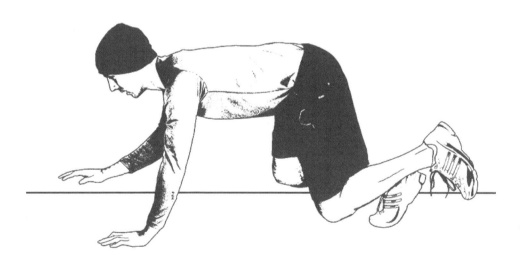

Quadrupedal Movement

- Get on the ground—on all fours in the classic "quadruped" position.
- Keep your back horizontal as you scuttle forward along the ground.
- Try to coordinate your opposite arm and leg to move in unison.
- Be careful not to skin your palms or knees on rough concrete.

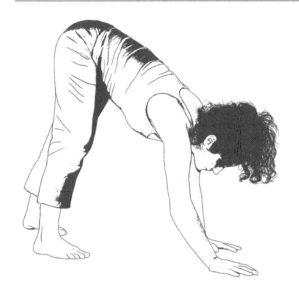

Bear Walk

- Begin in the quadruped position, with your butt elevated in the air.
- Walk your arms and leg forward, keeping your knees as straight as possible.
- Move one leg, then one arm in a slow forward "loping" motion.

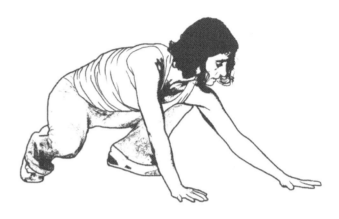

Kangaroo Walk

- Assume a low squat on the floor, with your pelvis angled so one foot is in front of the other.
- Reach your hands forward to make contact with the ground.
- Shift the weight into your palms and hop your legs forward, maintaining the angled position of your hips.
- *Make it harder:* Increase your speed so you gallop across the floor.

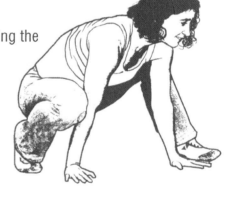

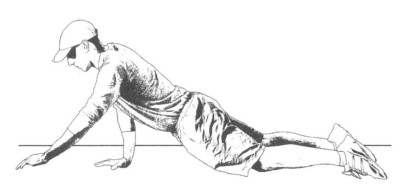

Leg Drag

- Start in the "upward dog" yoga posture.
- Pull yourself forward along the ground, using just upper body strength.
- Your legs should feel like deadweight behind you.
- Place a towel under your feet to prevent shredding your shoes.

Backward Leg Drag

- Get on the floor with your chest facing the ceiling and your legs extended in front of you.
- Reach your hands behind you and lift your bottom from the floor.
- Start moving your hands so you drag yourself backward, balancing on your heels.

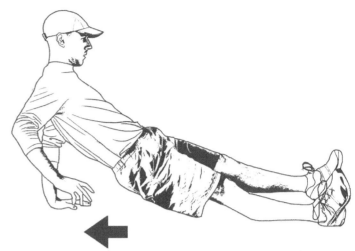

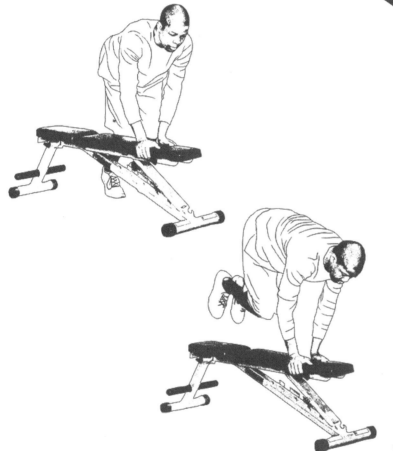

Lateral Bench Hops

- Place your hands on a bench or straddle a line on the ground.
- Hop from one side of the bench/line to the other side.
- Repeat back and forth, staying tight through your trunk and trying to keep your feet together.
- *Make it harder:* Do it on one leg!

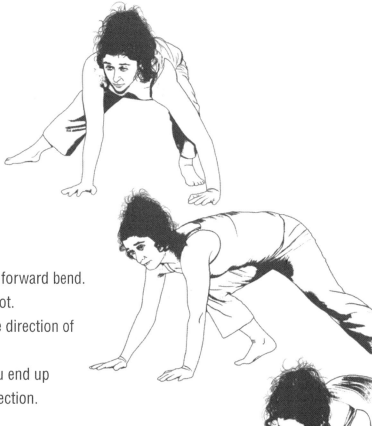

Side Crawl

- Begin in a low, wide-legged forward bend.
- Reach both hands to one foot.
- Lift your legs and hop in the direction of your hands.
- Repeat the steps so that you end up moving sideways in one direction.

Crab Walk

- Get on all fours with your chest and belly facing upwards.
- Keep your bottom off the ground while you walk your feet and hands forward like a crab.
- *Variation:* Move backward and sideways to work different muscle groups.

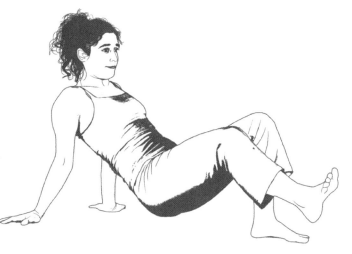

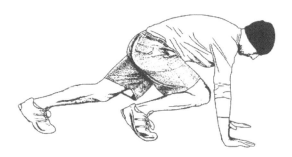

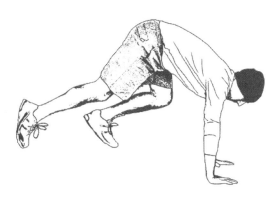

Mountain Climbers

- Start in a quadruped position with one leg forward near your hands.
- Explode through your legs, switching the position of your feet
- Try to bring your feet as far forward as you can with each cycle.
- Stay in one place; you shouldn't move forward.

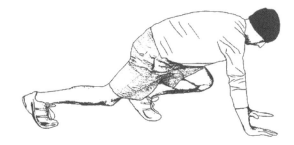

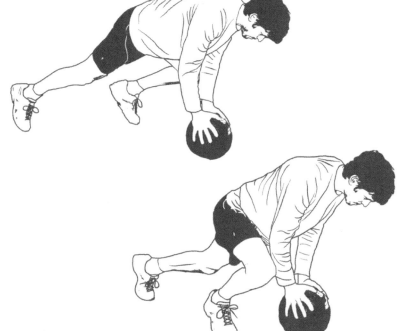

Med Ball Mountain Climber

- Perform the same basic motion as the mountain climber.
- Rather than having your hands on the ground, place them on a medicine ball.
- Focus on balance and core engagement.

Single Leg Mountain Climber

- Do the same basic motion as with a regular mountain climber.
- Hop forward and backward on one leg instead of two.

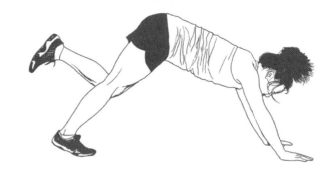

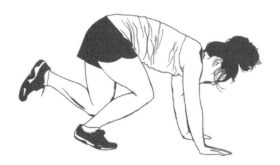

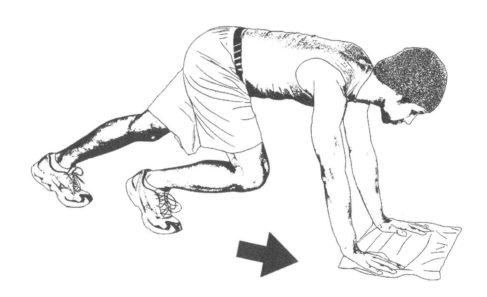

Towel Push

- Assume a high plank position, and place both hands on a towel.
- Keep your arms and shoulders tight.
- Push forward with your legs to propel yourself along the ground.
- *Variation:* Push an ab wheel or barbell with weights rather than the towel.

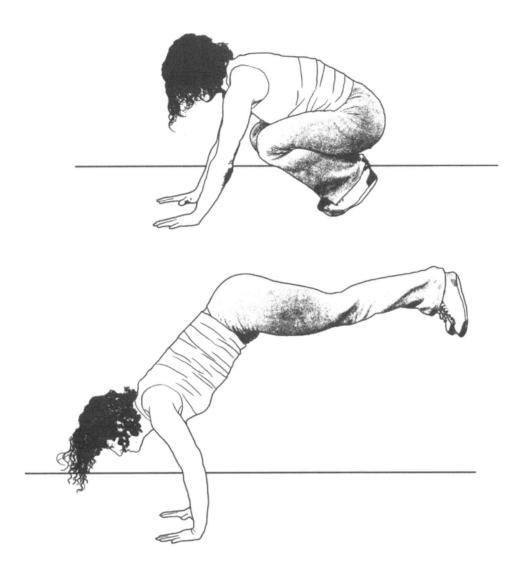

Donkey Kick

• Begin on the floor in a low crouch with your weight spread evenly between your hands and feet.

• Shift your weight forward onto your hands and explode your lower body upward into the air.

• Kick your legs behind you like a mule or donkey.

• Tuck you knees under your body as you return to the starting position.

Chapter 2

"Strong legs are the foundation of any serious athlete and should be pursued feverishly in your workout design."

Pillars of Steel

Strong legs: Who doesn't want them? Let's see—they allow you to run, leap, climb, bike, and are critical in practically every other sports activity that you can imagine. Aside from the fact that skinny jeans look a tad awkward on muscular thighs, there is really no reason that you shouldn't aim to increase your leg strength. Strong legs are the foundation of any serious athlete and should be pursued feverishly in your workout design.

You need strong legs!

When our aim is to build leg strength, it's natural to gravitate to a few fundamental movement categories. The general groupings that you'll find listed in this chapter include the following elements:

- **Squats:** Fixing your feet to the ground and lowering your hips/pelvis toward the floor.

- **Lunges:** Stepping away from a basic stance and catching your weight with the leg.

- **Deadlifts:** Picking items off the floor while hinging forward from the waist.

- **Step-ups:** Placing a foot on an elevated surface and then lifting your body up to that level.

- **Calf Raises:** Pushing through the balls of your feet in order to lift your heels off the floor.

- **Jumps:** Explosive movements yielding air time!

As you follow along, attempting skills from the basic movement groupings, you will probably notice that certain muscle groups tend to take the bulk of the punishment. The muscle groups that are targeted are those that will have the greatest impact on your athletic performance. Here are the lucky few:

- **Glutes:** The big muscle mass on your tail end; aka the "junk in your trunk." Their main function is to extend your hips, assisting with squats, deadlifts, jumps, and step-ups.

- **Quads:** Those mighty thigh muscles—think of the tree trunks exhibited by professional bike racers or alpine skiers. These muscles work to straighten your knee for basically all of the same motions listed above.

- **Hamstrings:** The oft-forgotten group found hiding from the seat of your pants to behind your knees. They flex the knee and help to extend the hip. You'll feel them in bridging and curling motions as well as with deadlifts and step-ups.

- **Calves:** The bulbous little guys that give shape to the back of your lower legs. They are the prime mover for lifting the heels off the ground and come into play with many explosive/power moves.

Students of anatomy will quickly spot a few deficiencies in this list. What about the hip flexors, adductor group, or hip rotators? How come we're missing the ankle dorsiflexors, evertors, or toe movers?

It's not that those muscle groups aren't important. They are. Just ask any physical therapist.

The reason that they're missing from this section is simple: Your athletic performance will be maximized if you put most of your focus on the muscle groups listed above. Time is precious. Instead of spinning your wheels targeting every single one of the 600+ muscles of your body, focusing on the big groups that provide the most power is the best use of your workout time.

The obvious caveat is that if you find yourself frequently injured, in pain, or suffering from poor stability, it would be a smart idea to consult with an exercise specialist. Addressing deficiencies in your smaller muscle groups has its place in training, but that is a topic best covered in a discussion of prehab. Let's save it for another book!

Enough yapping.

It's time for a Squat Fest!

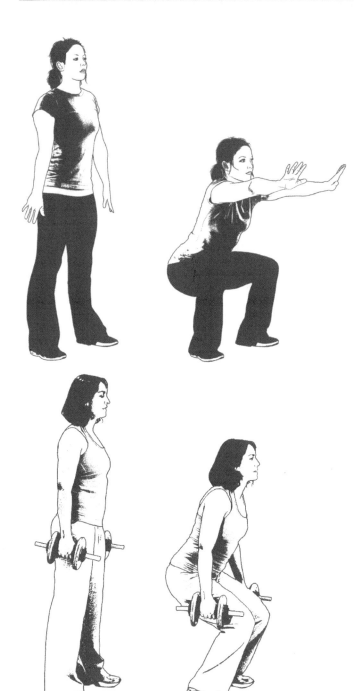

Air Squat

- Stand with your feet positioned at hip-width or slightly wider.
- Let your feet rotate out slightly.
- Drop your bottom backward, and counterbalance with your arms swinging forward.
- Don't let your knees turn inward.

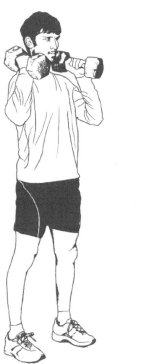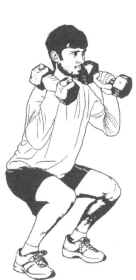

Dumbbell Squat

- Do the same basic motion as an air squat, but hold two dumbbells by your hips.
- Try to spread your weight evenly from your toes to your heels.
- Go as far as you can without losing your natural lumbar curve.

Dumbbell Front Squat

- Raise two dumbbells to shoulder height, keeping your elbows elevated.
- Squat down while engaging your core musculature to avoid lateral sway/rotation.

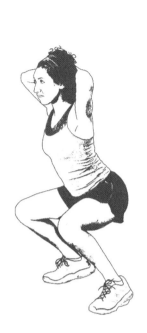
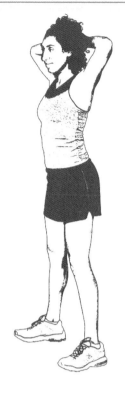

Prisoner Squat

- Perform a basic body-weight squat, but keep your hands interlaced behind your head.
- This position forces more mid-thoracic engagement.
- Try to keep your shoulder blades pulled back and downward along your spine.

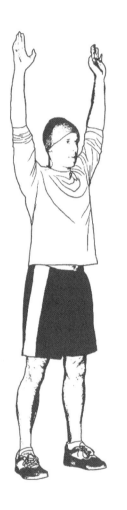
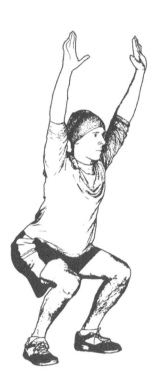

Overhead Squat

- Stand with your feet spread shoulder-width apart and raise your arms overhead.
- Lower into a squat, while pulling your shoulder blades together and keeping your arms above you.

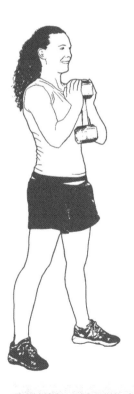
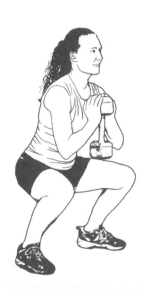

Goblet Squat

- Hold a single dumbbell at chest height by squeezing the bell between your palms.
- Fire your lateral glute muscles to actively spread your knees.

Plate Squat

- Stand with your feet shoulder-width apart and hug a weight plate to your chest with both arms.
- Lower into a squat and go as far as you can before returning to stand.
- Don't let your back lose its neutral alignment.

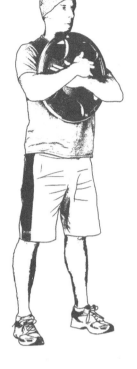
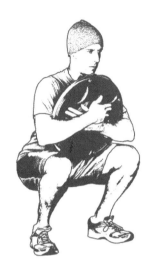

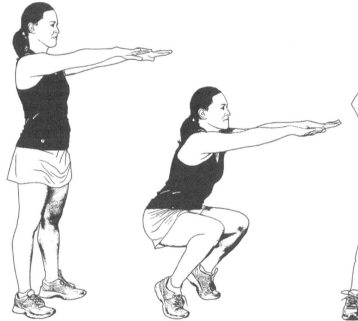

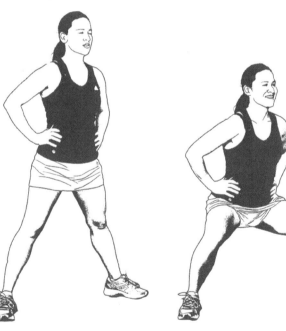

Tiptoe Squat

- Drop down to a squat while simultaneously rocking forward onto your toes.
- Try to stay balanced on your toes as you stand up to the starting position.
- *Make it harder*: Stay balanced on your tiptoes as you ascend and lower through multiple squats.

Sumo Squat

- Spread your feet double shoulder-width apart with feet rotated outward.
- Lower to a squat while being careful to prevent your knees from caving inward.

Split Squat

- Place one foot forward, approximately one step length ahead.
- Drop down into a split squat.
- Let the heel of your back leg peel off the floor.
- Try to keep your pelvis level.

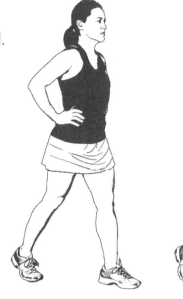
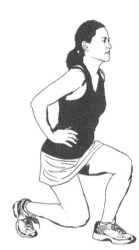

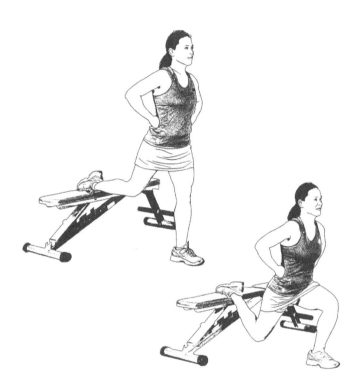

Bulgarian Split Squat

- Put your back leg up onto a bench or chair.
- Hop the front foot forward a few inches.
- Drop down into a squat, watching that your front leg doesn't veer inward.

Elevated Front Foot Split Squat

- Place your front leg on a stair or small box.
- Lower your body into the split squat position.
- Return to the elevated position.
- *Variation:* Hold a medicine ball or dumbbells for extra resistance.

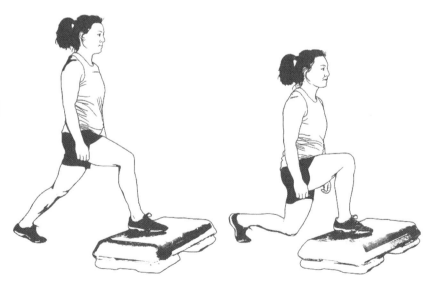

Squat Hold

- Spread your feet shoulder-width apart.
- Lower into a squat.
- Go as far as you can without losing your lumbar spine curvature.
- Keep weight distributed evenly from heel to toes.
- Hold for time.

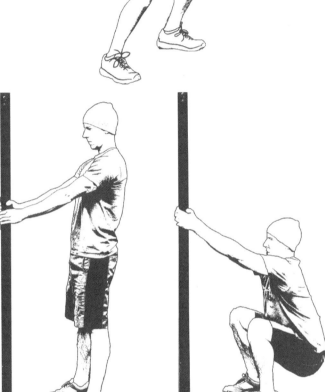

Assisted Squat

- Stand with your feet shoulder-width apart and grasp a vertical bar with your hands.
- Lower yourself down into a deep squat while holding the bar for support.
- Allow yourself to go lower than you could if not supported.
- Return to standing using your hands for light assist if needed.
- *Make it harder:* Try it on just one leg.

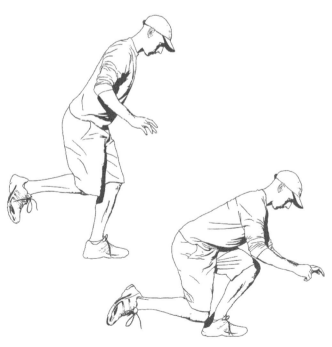

Crouched Single Leg Squat

- Balance on one leg with the opposite leg held slightly off the ground behind you.
- Lower into a single leg squat, watching that your knee doesn't deviate inward/outward.
- Go as far as you can without losing your balance.
- Return to standing.

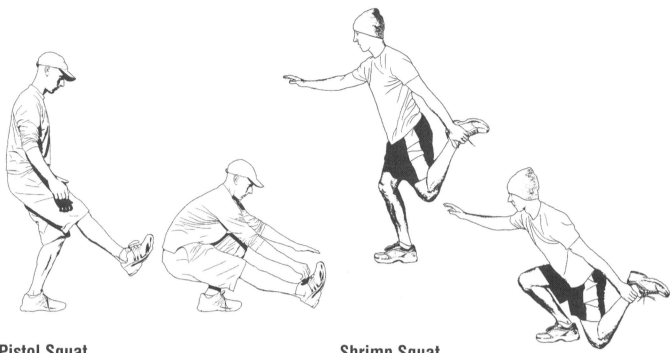

Pistol Squat

- Balance on a single leg, with the other leg held in front of your body.
- Lower down to a single leg squat, using the opposite leg as a counterweight.
- Use good control and try not to bounce.
- *Variation:* Hold a dumbbell or medicine ball for extra resistance.

Shrimp Squat

- Begin like a Crouched Single Leg Squat, but hold the ankle of your elevated leg behind you.
- Lower carefully to nearly touch your back knee to the floor and then stand up.
- Use your free hand as a counterweight.
- Be conscious of safe knee alignment.

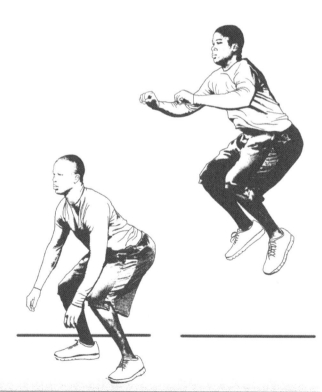

Squat Jump

- Start with your feet spread shoulder-width apart and your trunk tipped forward some.
- Lower to a partial squat then explode upward with a strong jump.
- Land softly, sucking up the ground with your feet.
- *Make it harder:* Add a tuck (grabbing your knees) at the top of your jump.

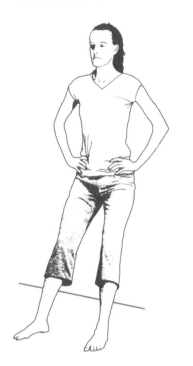
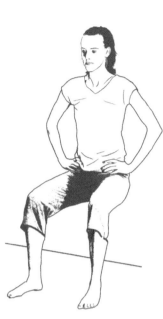

Wall Slide

- Place your feet approximately 18 inches away from a wall.
- Lower yourself backward, and support yourself on the wall.
- Lower to a squat, at least 90 degrees at your knees.
- Press upward to the starting position and repeat.

Wall Sit

- Perform the same beginning movement as the Wall Slide but stay down in the squat.
- Hold for time staying at a 90 degree angle at your knees.
- Don't let your knees cave in or outward.

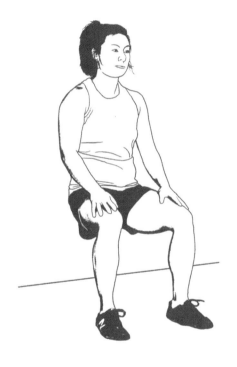

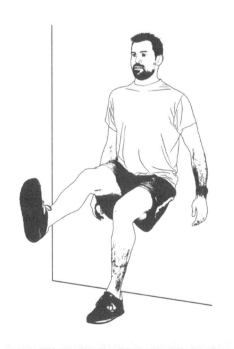

Single Leg Wall Sit

- Start in the same position as the Wall Sit, squatting 90 degrees at your knees.
- Lift one leg off the floor, trying to extend your knee fully.
- Balance in a single leg squat, resting against the wall.
- Watch the alignment of your weight bearing leg.
- Hold for time.

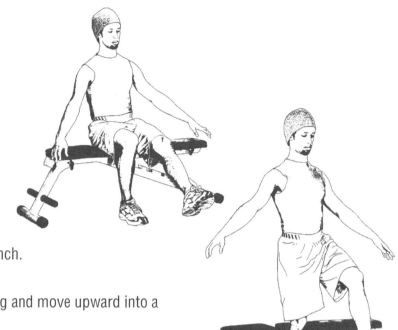

Single Leg Get-up

- Sit on a low chair, plyo box, or weight bench.
- Hold one leg a few inches off the floor.
- Push forcefully through your grounded leg and move upward into a standing position.
- Lower down on the single leg and repeat.
- *Make it harder:* Hold a weight plate for extra resistance.

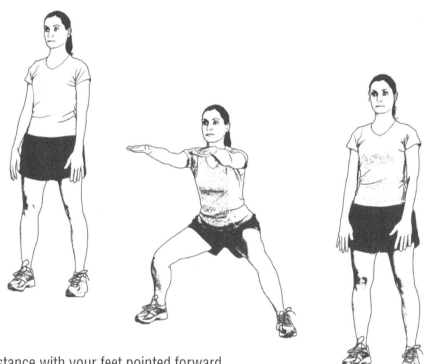

Side Step Squat

- Begin in a regular stance with your feet pointed forward.
- Step out to the side while simultaneously dropping to a deep squat.
- Raise your hands for counterbalance as needed.
- As you stand upward, bring the second leg to meet the first, so that you move sideways across the floor.

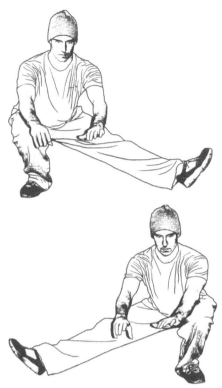

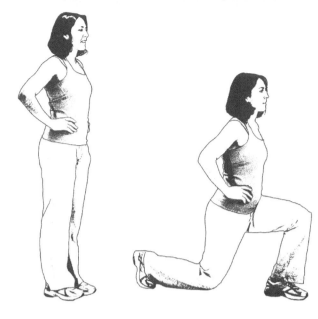

Forward Lunge

- Stand tall with your hands resting on your hips.
- Take a large step forward, and accept the weight onto your front leg.
- Lower your weight onto the front leg, allowing your knee to bend.
- Don't let your knee drop inward.
- Push hard through the front leg to propel yourself back to the starting position.

Cossack Squat

- Stand with your feet approximately double shoulder-width apart.
- Shift your weight to one leg and lower down into a deep squat over that leg.
- Rock onto the heel of your other foot with your leg extended and toes pointed to the ceiling.
- Carefully shift your weight to obtain the squat position over the other leg.
- *Variation:* Stand up completely before switching squat positions.

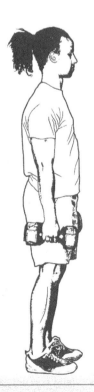

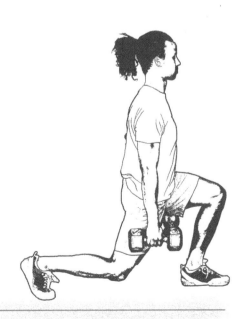

Dumbbell Forward Lunge

- Perform a basic Forward Lunge, holding two dumbbells for resistance.
- Mix it up by holding just one dumbbell at a time by your side.
- *Variation:* Hold the dumbbells in the racked position at your shoulders.

Prisoner Lunge

- Use the same Forward Lunge motion, except keep your hands interlaced on the back of your head.
- This position forces more upper back and shoulder girdle activation.

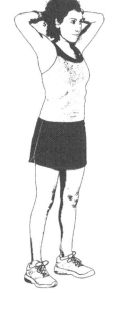
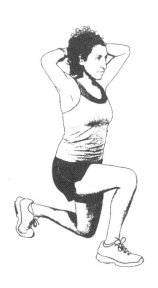

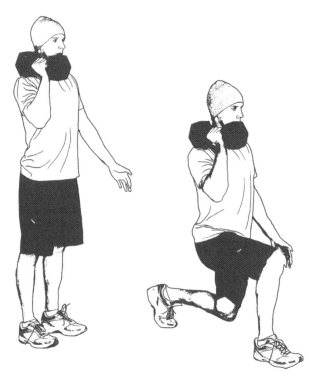

Offset Dumbbell Lunge

- Hold a single dumbbell at your shoulder height.
- Step forward on the same side as the dumbbell, dropping into lunge.
- Return to the starting position and repeat.
- Focus on staying tight through your core so that the offset weight doesn't make you unsteady.

Side Lunge

- Stand with your legs spread shoulder-width apart and your hands resting on your hips.
- Take a large step to the side, transferring weight onto the moving leg.
- Lowering carefully into a deep knee bend.
- Don't let your foot rotate too far outward, and pay attention to safe knee alignment.

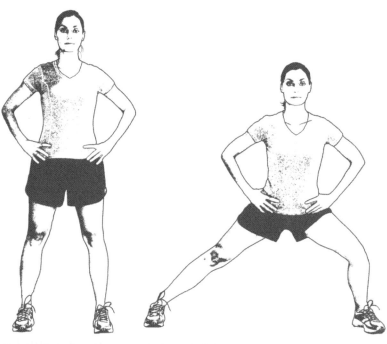

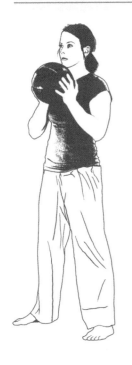
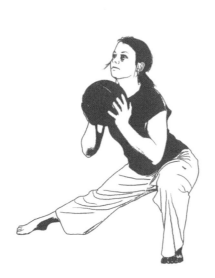

Resisted Side Lunge

- Perform the same basic Side Lunge movement, but hold a medicine ball or dumbbells as resistance.
- Drop as far as you can without losing your spinal curve or causing knee discomfort.

Walking Lunge

- Clear a path to move forward along the ground.
- Keep your hands on your hips or elevated on your head.
- Walk forward, dropping to a deep lunge on each step.
- Try to touch your knee to the ground on each step.
- Avoid an extra side-to-side motion.

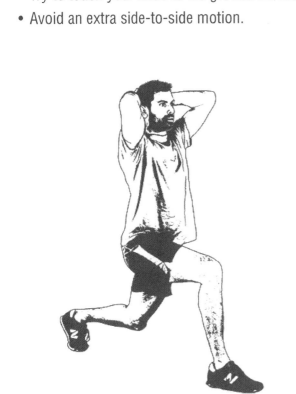
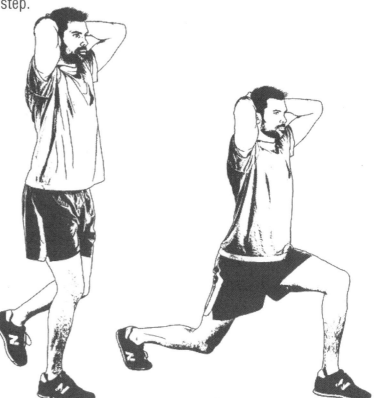

Bridge

- Lie on the floor with your knees bent and feet placed on the ground waist-width apart.
- Tighten your abdominal muscles and push through your feet to lift your bottom.
- Drive your hips as high as you can while actively spreading your knees.

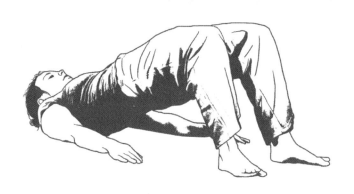

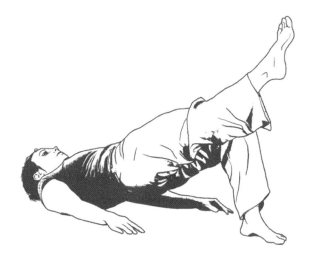

Single Leg Bridge

- Begin in the bridge position with one foot elevated off the ground.
- Press through your bottom leg, lifting your hips off the floor.
- Stay tight through your core so that you don't rotate.
- Keep your knee from dropping inward.

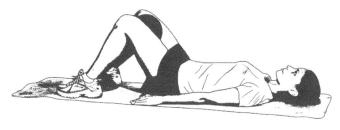

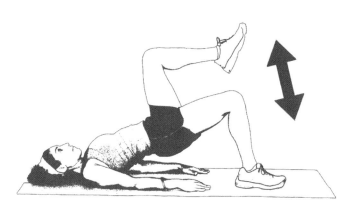

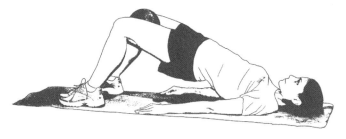

Marching Bridge

- Lift your hips off the floor in the basic Bridge position.
- Lift one knee upward, raising your foot off the ground.
- Lower that leg, and then lift the other so that you "march" your knees up and down.
- Protect your back by keeping your abs contracted.

Bridge & Ball Squeeze

- Assume the bottom position of a Bridge, and place a medicine ball between your knees.
- Squeeze the ball firmly between your thighs, and then press through your feet to lift into the upward bridge position.

Body-weight Hamstring Curl

- Lie on the floor with a towel under your feet.
- Drive your hips upward, lifting you bottom off the floor.
- Slide your heels toward your bottom while allowing your knees to bend.
- Lower smoothly and repeat back and forth.

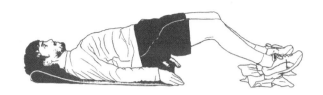

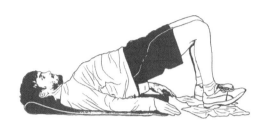

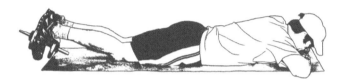

Dumbbell Hamstring Curl

- Lie face-down on your belly.
- Hold a dumbbell between your feet.
- Tighten your hamstrings to raise the weight up toward your trunk.
- Lower the dumbbell and repeat.

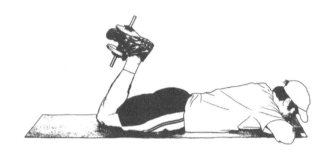

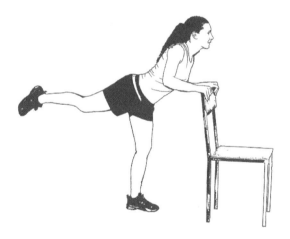

Bent Over Hamstring Curl

- Bend over at your waist, holding a chair or wall for support.
- Extend one leg behind your body.
- Lift your heel toward your rear end and lower it slowly to the extended position.
- Make it harder: Use an ankle weight or have a partner provide manual resistance.

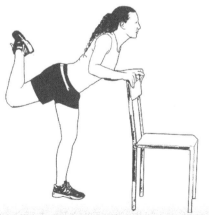

Double Leg Hip Extension

- Lie on your back with your feet placed on top of a weight bench or small plyo box.
- Squeeze your glutes and drive your hips upward.
- Stay tight through your trunk to protect your back.
- Lower slowly and repeat.

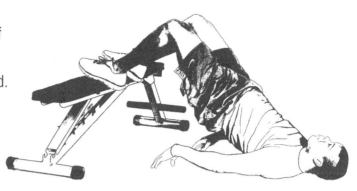

Single Leg Hip Exttension

- Start in the same position as the exercise above, but hold one foot elevated off the bench.
- Drive through your bottom foot to lift your waist in the air.
- Focus on the stability of your hip and knee to avoid any lateral rocking.

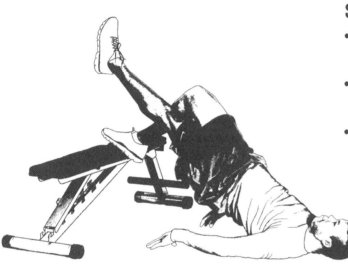

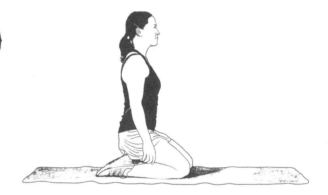

Kneeling Hip Thrust

- Kneel on the floor with your bottom resting on your heels.
- Tighten your quads and glutes to lift your bottom and elevate your trunk higher.
- Lower back to the starting position.
- *Make it harder*: Hold a weight plate for resistance or try to explode off the floor and bring your feet forward to assume a squat position.

Glute Lift

- Get on the floor on your hands and knees.
- Lift one foot off the floor while keeping your knee bent.
- Fire your glute to extend the hip and raise the leg upward.
- *Make it harder:* Use an ankle weight or have a partner provide extra resistance.

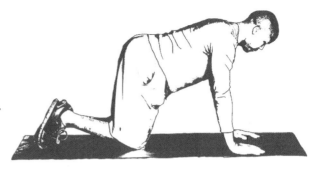

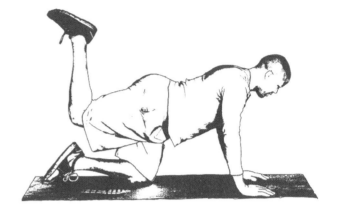

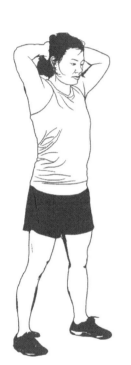

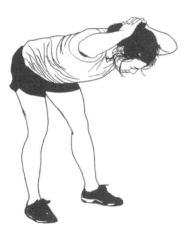

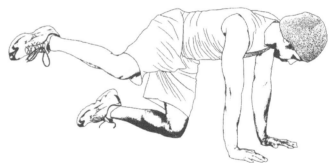

Good Morning

- Stand with your feet shoulder-width apart and your hands placed on your head.
- Hinge forward from your waist, dropping your trunk into a bow.
- Only go as far as you can without losing your lumbar curve.
- Tighten your glutes and hamstrings, while driving forward through your hips, to bring yourself to a standing position.

Fire Hydrant Leg Raise

- Get on your hands and knees.
- Raise one leg to the side, imitating a dog peeing on a fire hydrant.
- Lower slowly and repeat.
- Try to isolate the movement to your hip rather than letting your trunk rotate.

Single Leg Good Morning

- Balance on one leg with your hands raised near your head.
- Hinge forward from your waist while letting the back leg rise as a counterweight.
- Drop your chest as far as you can without rounding your low back.
- Return to the upright position on one leg and repeat.

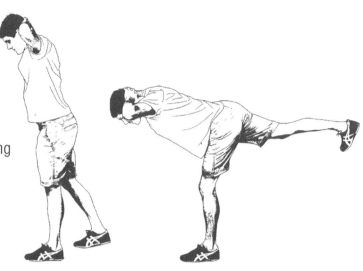

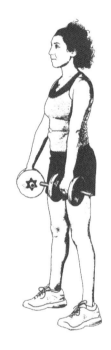

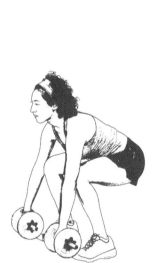

Dumbbell Deadlift

- Position your feet shoulder-width apart with your feet in a slight outward rotation.
- Bend your knees and drop your hips low enough so that you can grasp a pair of dumbbells from the floor.
- Push through the ground, driving your knees straight and hips forward to return to a standing position.
- Lower and repeat.
- *Variation:* Lift a medicine ball.

Dumbbell Stiff Leg Deadlift

- Begin with your feet shoulder-width apart.
- Hinge forward from your hips, bending as far as you can without losing your lumbar curve.
- Allow your knees to bend slightly as needed to maintain spine alignment.
- Pick the dumbbells off the floor, stand tall, lower and repeat.

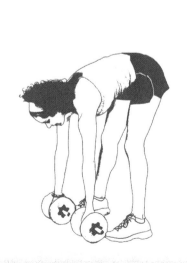

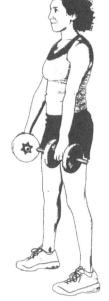

Dumbbell Sumo Deadlift

- Spread your legs nearly double shoulder-width with your legs rotated outward in a "sumo stance."
- Bend forward to pick up a dumbbell.
- Drive your hips forward as you lift your back and stand tall.
- Lower the dumbbell and repeat.

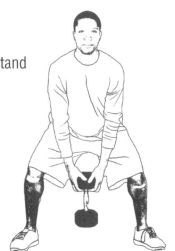
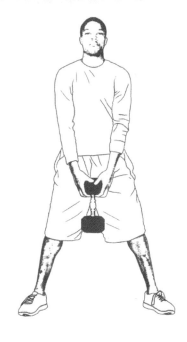

Dumbbell Suitcase Deadlift

- Assume a shoulder-width stance with a single dumbbell at your side.
- Squat down as if you were picking up a suitcase.
- Don't let either knee collapse inward and don't allow significant trunk rotation.
- Drive through your glutes and quads to stand up.
- Repeat with multiple repetitions on each side.

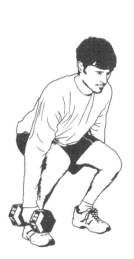
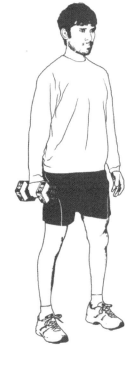

Bench Step-up

- Place one foot on a sturdy weight bench with your toes pointed forward or slightly outward.
- Shift your weight onto the elevated foot, push hard through your leg, and rise upward on the bench.
- Straighten your knee fully then lower back to the floor.
- *Make it harder:* Add a small jump at the top, so the movement becomes plyometric.

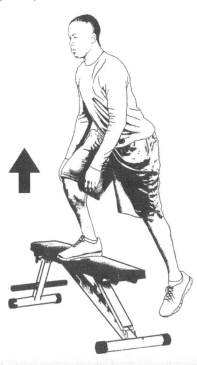

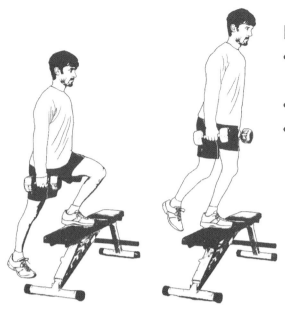

Dumbbell Step-up

- Perform the same basic Bench Step-up listed above, but hold one or two dumbbells for extra resistance.
- Rise up and lower on the same leg for maximal effort.
- Either alternate legs on each repetition or do multiple reps on one leg (harder).

Side Step-up

- Use a stair or small box for this exercise.
- Stand sideways against the stair, and place one foot top with the toes pointed forward.
- Shift your weight laterally, and lift yourself into full extension.
- Try to keep your pelvis level.
- *Make it harder:* Hold a dumbbell or weight plate.

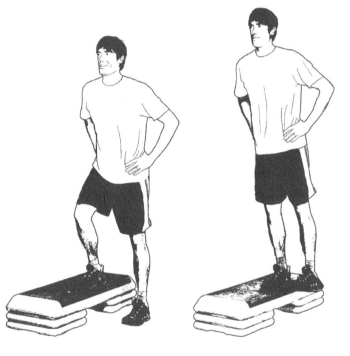

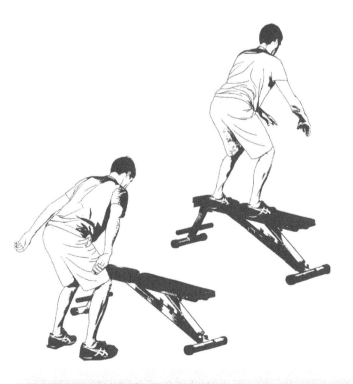

Bench Jump

- Face off with a bench approximately 1–2 feet in front of you.
- Perform a partial squat then explode upward to jump and land on top of the bench.
- Hop off and land softly.
- *Make it harder:* Hold a medicine ball for resistance.

Calf Raise

- Start in a natural stance with your heels a few inches apart.
- Rise upward on your tiptoes, contracting your calf musculature to the full extent.
- Descend slowly and repeat, working a full range of motion on each rep.

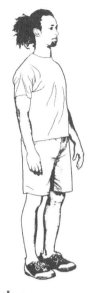
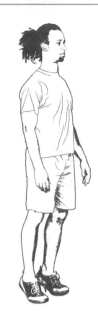

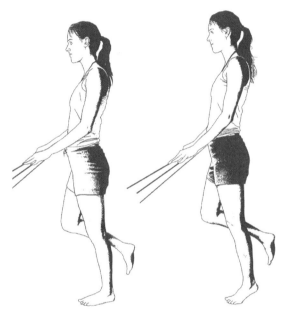

Single Leg Calf Raise

- Balance on a single leg, holding a rail or wall for support as needed.
- Raise your body weight onto the toes of your grounded foot.
- Move through the full range of motion and lower slowly.
- Work a variety of angles, letting the ankle roll inward and outward as able.

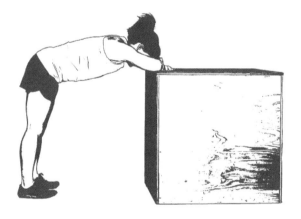

Donkey Calf Raise

- Bend forward from your waist, supporting your trunk on your forearms (on a box or countertop).
- Rise upward on the tiptoes of both feet as high as you can.
- *Variation:* Do it like a bodybuilder and have a partner sit on your pelvis (be careful!).

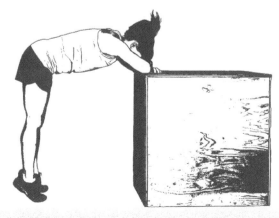

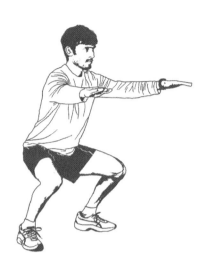
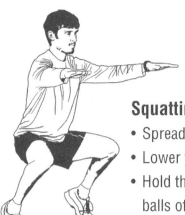

Squatting Calf Raise

- Spread your legs at least shoulder-width apart.
- Lower your hips to a medium depth squat.
- Hold the squat and shift your weight forward to the balls of your feet.
- Rise upward on your tiptoes.
- Lower and repeat.
- *Make it harder:* Hold dumbbells for resistance.

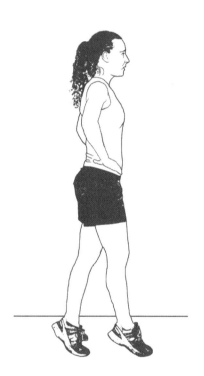

Tiptoe Walking

- Tighten your calves and lift yourself up onto your tiptoes.
- Stay balanced on your tiptoes and walk forward for time or distance.
- *Make it harder:* Hold dumbbells or a medicine ball for resistance.

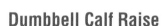

Dumbbell Calf Raise

- Same basic motion as a regular Calf Raise, but hold dumbbells at sides for resistance.
- *Variation:* Hold a single dumbbell at shoulder height or overhead to challenge core strength and stability.

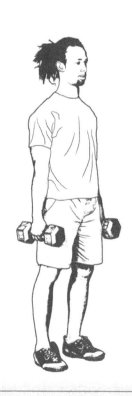
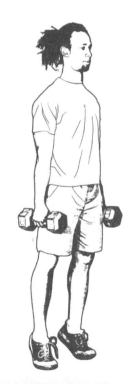

Seated Dumbbell Calf Raise

- Sit on a bench and place the balls of your feet on a stack of weight plates so your heels are free.
- Hold one or two dumbbells on your knees.
- Press through the balls of your feet to lift your heels.
- Move through as much range of motion as possible.

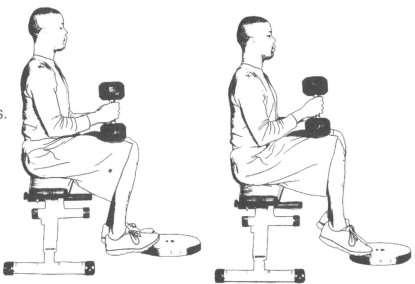

Broad Jump

- Identify two lines on the ground spread multiple feet apart.
- Stand behind one line, drop to a slight squat, and then explode forward.
- Try to jump past the second line.
- Land softly, striking with your forefeet first.

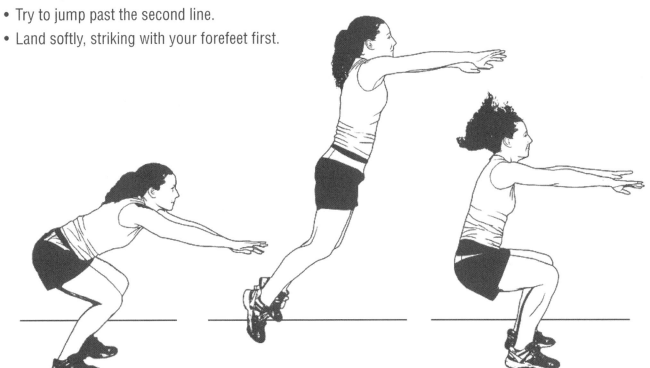

Split Jump

- Start with one foot placed 18–24 inches in front of the other foot.
- Jump upward and switch the position of your feet in the air.
- Land softly, and then explode up again switching your feet back and forth.
- *Variation:* Hold your hands at your waist or behind your head.

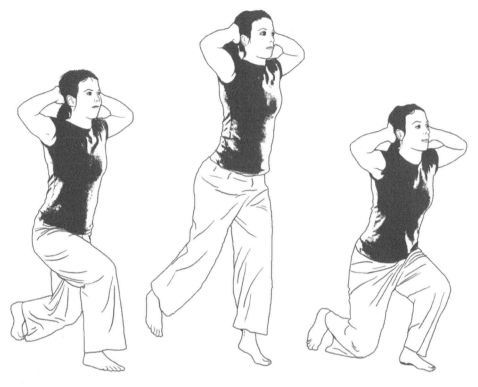

Resisted Split Jump

- Make the Split Jumps more strenuous by holding a medicine ball, weight plate, or dumbbells for resistance.

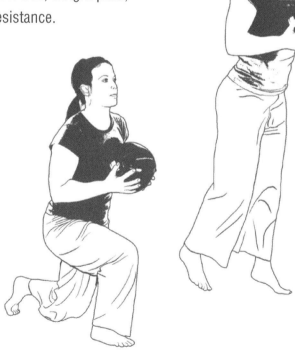
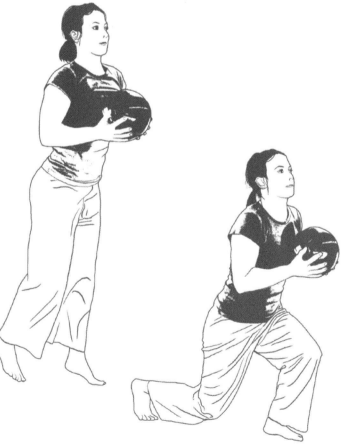

Single Leg Jump

- Balance on a single leg.
- Drop to a partial squat, and then explode upward.
- Jump as high as you can then land softly.
- Protect your knee by being aware of its alignment.
- *Variation:* Go for distance, doing a single leg broad jump.

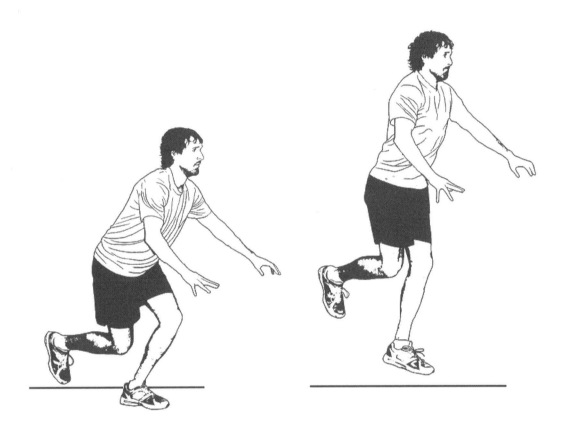

Chapter 3

"A muscular upper body allows better performance in everything from basic survival to your favorite weekend sports."

Gorilla Arms

Do you value your ability to pull yourself to safety from a cliff's edge? Or hurl something heavy at a predator? Or simply help grandpa off the floor? What about popping-up onto your surfboard, passing a football, or grappling with your cousins at a family reunion?

Weak arms won't let you do that stuff.

A muscular upper body allows better performance in everything from basic survival to your favorite weekend sports. The greater your upper body strength, the better your performance will be, whatever activity you do.

This chapter is dedicated to sharing a selection of ways to build arm, shoulder, chest, and upper back strength.

If you already consider yourself a weight room veteran, then this section might be a bit of a refresher on ways to pump iron. Fear not. The coming chapters on barbells, kettlebells, and gymnastics-type strength should add more variety to your training repertoire.

For the sake of clarity, let's go over the definitions of a few basic movements.

- **Curls:** Any movement where you are flexing, or closing, the angle of a joint.

- **Extensions:** The opposite of a curl, in which you straighten, or open, the angle of a joint.

- **Raises:** Lifting a weight upward against gravity, typically with a straight arm.

- **Flies:** A type of raise, often performed across the body, meant to develop strength in your chest, shoulders, or back.

- **Presses:** A compound movement involving motion at two joints, where you push a weight away from your body.

- **Rows:** Another multi-joint movement that involves pulling a weight toward your body.

Where are the push-ups and pull-ups ?

Once you get into the chapter, you'll probably be surprised to see that these two body-weight movements are missing. With so many awesome push-up variations out there, I believe they warrant their own chapter. (For push-up movements, check out chapter 7, Mad Push-ups.) Likewise, pull-ups are fundamental to gymnastics strength, thus, you'll find all pull-up variations in chapter 8, Monkey Style.

What about grip strength?

You'll find that there are a few movements in this chapter that specifically target grip strength, but regrettably there isn't a huge selection. To strengthen the muscles that give you a vice-like grip you basically need to work on carrying, lifting, and holding onto heavy objects. Deadlifts and farmer walks will do this. Exercises that strengthen the wrist are helpful, as well as simply hanging from a bar.

Isolated, open-chain movements? What is this—the 1980s?

Don't hate. I'm with you 100%: Closed chain, compound movements are superior to single-joint weight lifting for a variety of reasons. Yet, for the purpose of an exercise encyclopedia, it is fair game to include them in here. Sometimes you might really have a need to strengthen one specific muscle. And, it's not like you'll be doing them every single workout. Given the breadth of skills in here, you'll likely only do them a few times per year in your workouts.

Here is an abbreviated list of muscles you'll be strengthening in this chapter. You'll see that, like in chapter 2, there are a few muscle groups that are not specifically targeted. Again, what you have is a distilled grouping meant to give you maximal return on your efforts.

- **Biceps:** These big guns bend your elbow bringing your forearm closer to your shoulder and are crucial to rows and arm "curling" motions.

- **Triceps:** Sitting quietly on the back of your arm, they function to straighten your elbow and are active during presses and elbow extensions.

- **Pecs:** Giving girth to your chest, the pecs sit on your rib cage and function to bring your arms in front of your body during presses and flies.

- **Deltoids:** Forming the spherical shape of your shoulder, the deltoids fire to lift your arms away from your body. You use them during raises and certain flies.

- **Trapezius:** Resting on your upper back, the traps function to move your shoulder blades. They get used during rows and shrugs.

You'll find that one of my favorite muscle groups, the latissimus dorsi, doesn't get much attention in this chapter. The lats pull your arms down to your body when they are in an elevated position and are thus critical in performing pull-ups. If you skip ahead to chapter 8, you'll find all kinds of creative ways to strengthen them.

Let's get to pumping some iron!

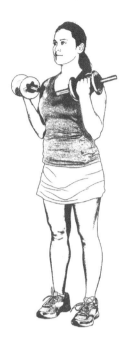
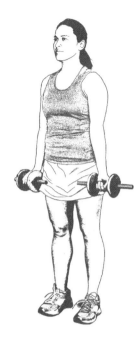

Bicep Curl

- Hold two dumbbells at your thighs.
- Flex your elbows and lift the weights to your shoulders.
- Lower weights back down to the starting position.

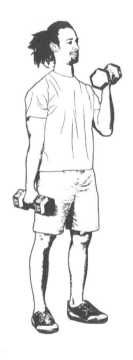
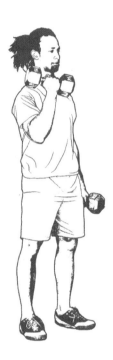

Alternating Bicep Curl

- Start with two dumbbells resting by your thighs.
- Curl one dumbbell to your chest, and then lower it back down.
- Repeat on the opposite side.
- Alternate curls from one side to the other.

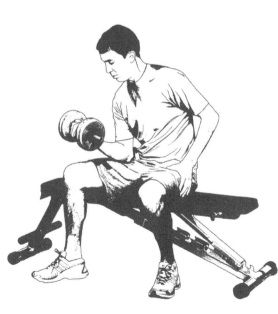

Concentration Curl

- Sit on a bench and hold one dumbbell, while supporting your elbow on your thigh.
- Curl the weight up and down, focusing on the quality of motion.
- *Variation:* Do the lift while standing in a partial squat, with your elbow supported on your thigh.

Single Arm Preacher Curl

- Place your elbow and upper arm on the cushion of an incline bench.
- Brace yourself with your opposite hand and an athletic foot placement.
- Curl a dumbbell from full elbow extension into full flexion.

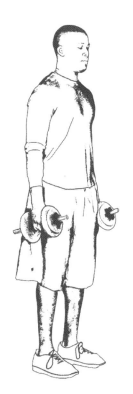
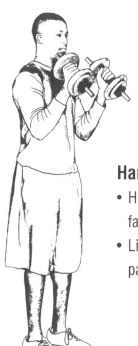
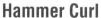

Hammer Curl

- Hold two dumbbells by your thighs with your palms facing inward.
- Lift the weights through a full curl but keep your palms facing each other.

Reverse Grip Bicep Curl

- Hold two dumbbells with your palms rotated downward or hold an E-Z bar (as shown in the picture).
- Keep your palms pointed to the floor as you curl the weights.

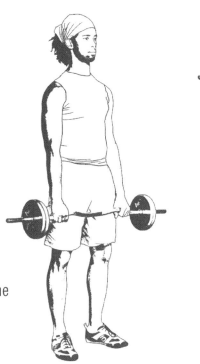
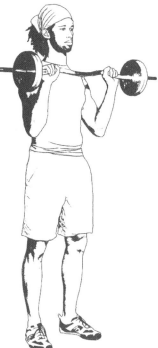

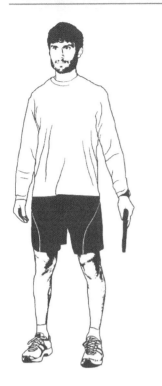 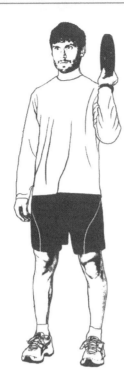

Plate Pinch Curl

- Hold a weight plate between your thumb and fingers.
- Begin with your hand by your side with your wrist in a neutral position.
- Lift the weight plate to your shoulder, using your fingertips to hold the plate.

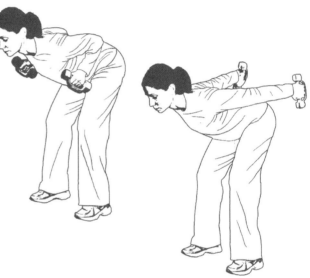

Bent Over Tricep Extension

- Bend over and hold two dumbbells by your chest.
- Straighten your arms to extend your elbows and lift the weights parallel with your back.
- Lower your hands, flexing your elbows back to the starting position.

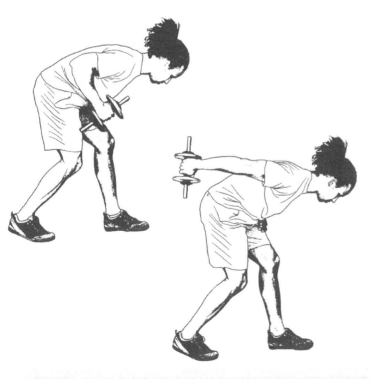

Tricep Kickback

- Bend forward at your waist, placing one hand on your thigh or a bench for support.
- Hold a single dumbbell by your chest.
- Straighten your elbow to lift the dumbbell behind you.
- Achieve full extension, pause, and then return to the chest.

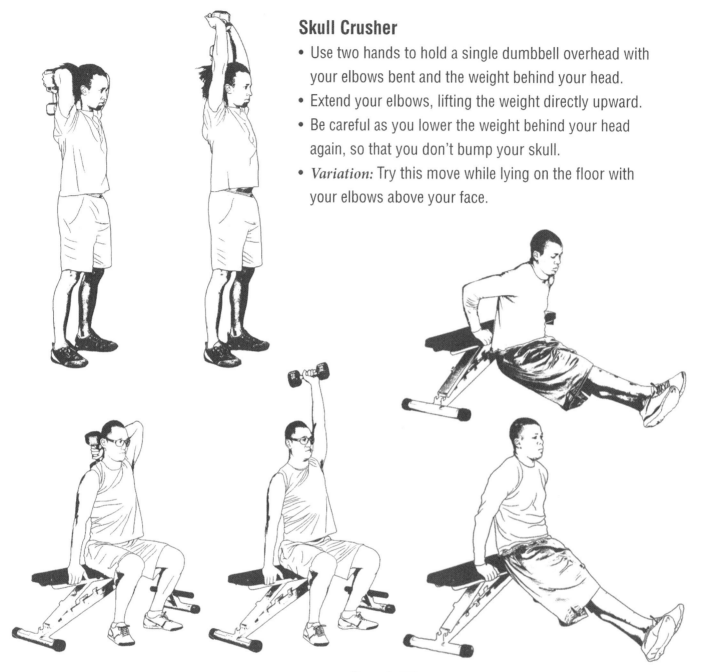

Skull Crusher

- Use two hands to hold a single dumbbell overhead with your elbows bent and the weight behind your head.
- Extend your elbows, lifting the weight directly upward.
- Be careful as you lower the weight behind your head again, so that you don't bump your skull.
- *Variation:* Try this move while lying on the floor with your elbows above your face.

Single Arm Skull Crusher

- Do the same basic motion as the Skull Crusher, but do it with just one arm.
- Strive to keep your elbow lifted the entire time.
- *Variation:* Vary sitting versus standing for different degrees of trunk support.

Bench Dip

- Place your palms on a bench with your fingers pointed forward.
- Extend your legs in front with your knees straight and heels on the ground.
- Lower your butt to the floor by bending your elbows, as in a "dipping" motion.
- Straighten your elbows to return to the starting position.
- *Make it harder:* Elevate your feet on another bench.

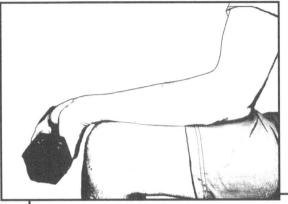

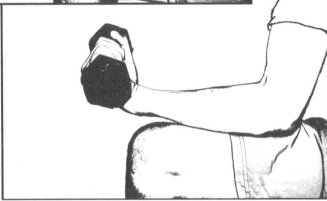

Wrist Curl

- Hold a dumbbell with your forearm supported on your thigh, palm facing the ceiling.
- Tighten your forearm to lift the weight upward against gravity, into full wrist flexion.
- Drop your wrist backward toward the floor again, returning to the starting position.

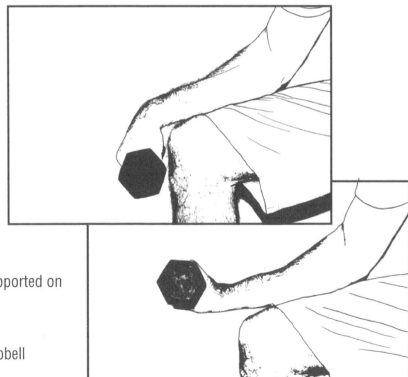

Reverse Wrist Curl

- Hold a dumbbell with your forearm supported on your thigh.
- Your palm should be facing the floor.
- Fire your wrist muscles to lift the dumbbell upwards.
- Isolate the motion to your wrist.

Wrist Roll-up

* Attach a 3-foot length of rope and weight plate to a short dowel.
* Straighten your arms in front of your body, keeping the dowel at chest height.
* Use wrist motion to rotate the dowel in one direction, wrapping the rope along the bar.
* Once the weight is fully elevated, reverse your wrist motion to lower it back to the floor.

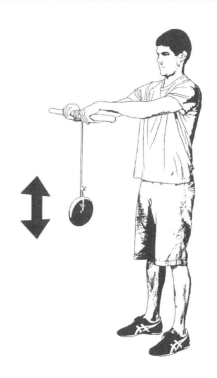

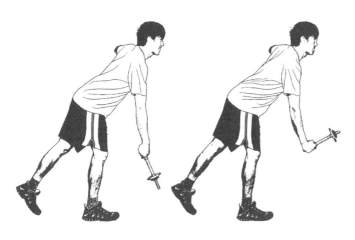

Resisted Radial Deviation

* Add weight to one side of an adjustable dumbbell.
* Hold the empty end of the dumbbell so that the weight is above your thumb.
* Keep your wrist in neutral alignment, and then lift the weight towards your shoulder without moving the rest of your arm.

Resisted Ulnar Deviation

* Use the same dumbbell configuration as with the Resisted Radial Deviation.
* Hold the empty end of the handle so that the weight is on the pinky-end of your hand.
* Move your wrist so that you raise the weight toward your trunk and then lower it away from you.

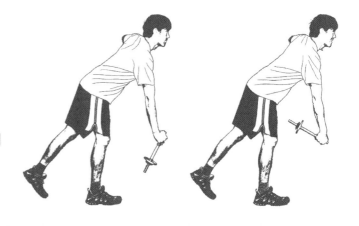

Hand Grip

- Hold a classic metal grip tool, a Gripmaster, or a stress ball.
- Squeeze your fingers to your palm.
- Hold for a few breaths, and then relax back into the open position.
- Try to avoid flexing your wrist inward.

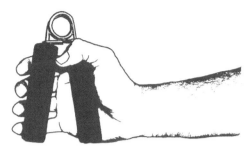

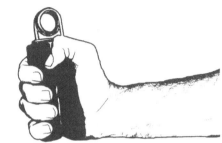

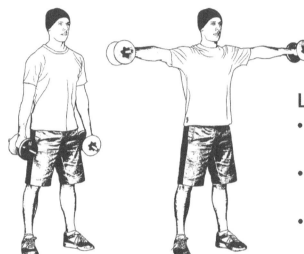

Lateral Raise

- Hold two dumbbells by your hips with your arms relaxed, elbows straight, and thumbs pointed forward.
- Tighten your trunk, fire your shoulders, and lift the weights directly sideways.
- Finish with your hands at about shoulder-height, and then lower to the starting position.

Forward Raise

- Hold a dumbbell with your arm straight and hand by your thigh.
- Lift the weight directly forward, stopping at shoulder-height.
- Keep your shoulder blade set back and down along your spine.
- *Variation:* Try lifting two dumbbells forward (one in each hand).

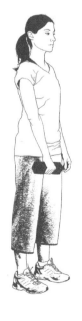

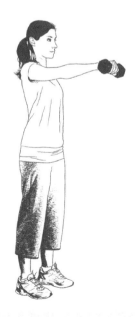

Weight Plate Forward Raise

- Use two hands to hold a weight plate in front of your pelvis.
- Raise the plate to shoulder-height, while keeping your elbows straight.
- Be careful to avoid hitting the weight against your pelvis as you lower it.

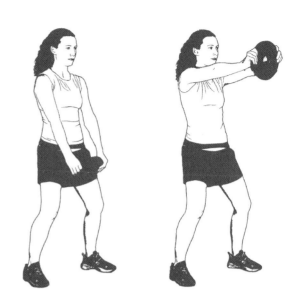

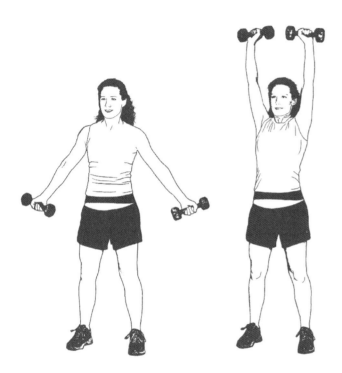

Overhead Lateral Raise

- Hold two dumbbells at your side with your thumbs pointed to the ceiling.
- Lift your arms outward to the side and stop once they are directly overhead.
- Raise and lower your hands as if making a snow angel.

Scapular-plane Raise

- Hold two dumbbells by your hips, with your wrists rotated outward slightly.
- Raise the weights on a plane of motion 30 to 45 degrees in front of your body.
- Stop once you achieve shoulder-height.
- Don't let your shoulders scrunch up to your ears: Keep your shoulder blades low on your back.

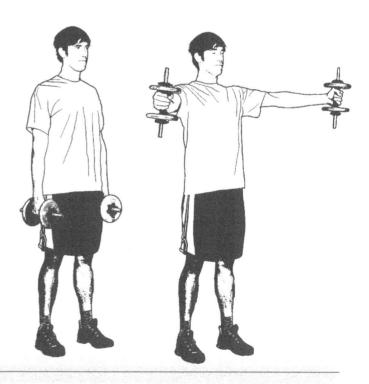

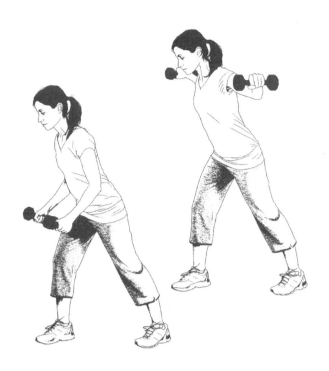

Bent Over Reverse Fly

- Hinge forward at your waist approximately 30 degrees while holding two dumbbells at your side.
- Try staggering your legs for balance.
- Raise the dumbbells backwards in a swinging motion as you pull your shoulder blades together.
- Stop at 90 degrees of elevation, and then lower to the starting position.

Single Arm Bent Over Reverse Fly

- Use a single arm for this Reverse Fly variation.
- Your opposite arm can rest on your leg for support.
- Try to make your shoulder blade glide back and inward along your rib cage as you lift your arm.

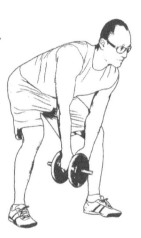

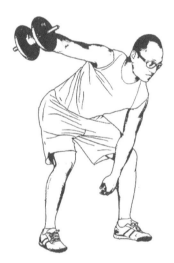

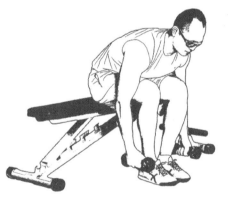

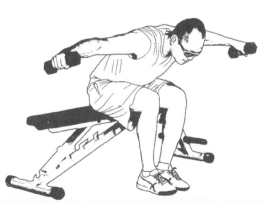

Seated Bent Over Reverse Fly

- Sit on a bench or chair to perform the basic Reverse Fly motion.
- Try supporting your abdomen on your thighs to allow greater focus on your posterior shoulder and mid-back muscles.

Supported Single Arm Reverse Fly

- This is the same basic concept as the Single Arm Reverse Fly, but use your opposite arm to support your trunk on a bench.
- Place your knee on the bench as well, to support your lower body, and bring your trunk into a nearly horizontal position.

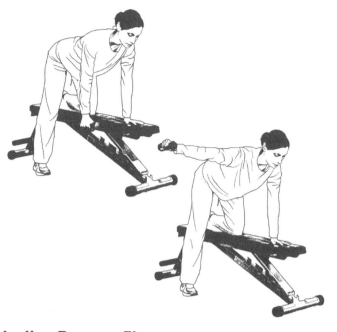

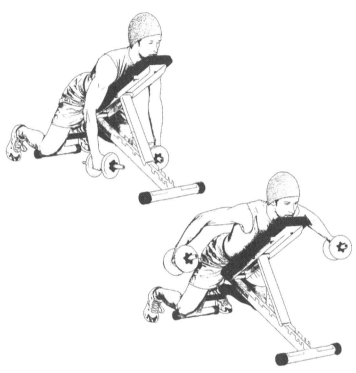

Incline Reverse Fly

- Position the backrest of a weight bench at a 45 degree angle.
- Rest your sternum on the cushion and let your arms hang to the floor.
- Pull your shoulder blades together and lift your arms out to the side.
- Stop when your hands are elevated to the height of your chest.

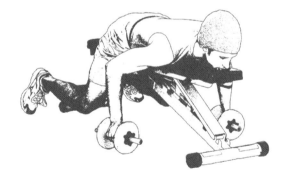

Prone Reverse Fly

- Lie on a flat weight bench with your chest and pelvis supported on the cushion.
- Perform the basic Reverse Fly motion, lifting your hands out to the side and level with your chest.

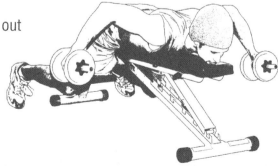

Side Lying Reverse Fly

- Lie on a bench with your body turned 90 degrees, so your side rests on the cushion.
- Hold a dumbbell with your top hand and start with it draped towards the floor.
- Raise the arm in an arc towards the ceiling, stopping when it is perpendicular to the floor.

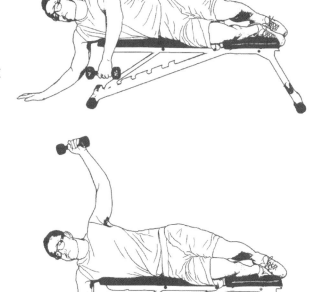

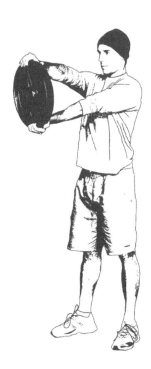

Truck Driver

- Hold a single weight plate with two hands.
- Lift the plate to shoulder-height and try to keep it there as long as possible.
- Rotate each hand from top to bottom, turning the plate as if you were driving a big truck.

Prone Shoulder External Rotation

- Lie on your belly on a bench, with one arm supported at a 90 degree angle from your body.
- Use shoulder rotation to raise a dumbbell from the floor to the level of your head.
- Reverse the rotation to lower the weight back down.

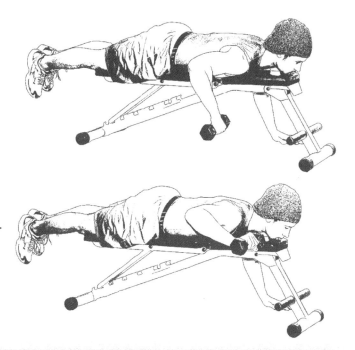

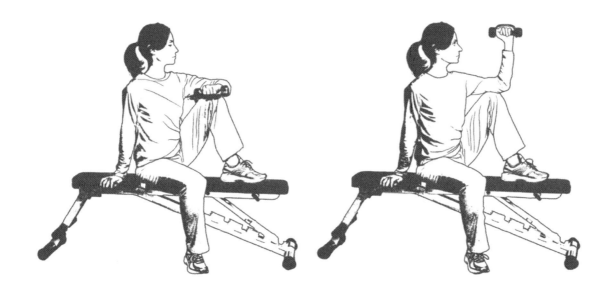

Seated Shoulder External Rotation

• Sit on a bench with your knee flexed and foot on the cushion.

• Place your elbow on your knee while holding a dumbbell at chest level.

• Rotate your hand to the ceiling using just a shoulder motion.

• Keep your elbow supported on the knee.

Scarecrow External Rotation

• Hold two dumbbells at your side with your elbows raised to shoulder-height.

• Your hands should be hanging to the floor and your elbows bent to 90 degrees.

• Use shoulder rotation to lift the weights to the ceiling.

• Keep your chest up and shoulders pulled backward.

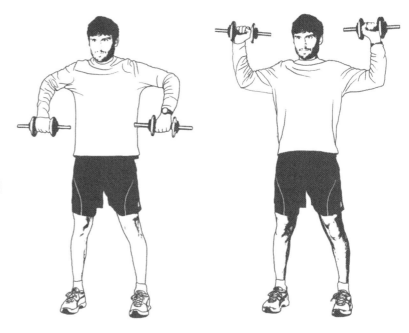

Lateral Raise & External Rotation

- Start with your hands by your hips, holding two dumbbells.
- Lift your arms to the height of your shoulders with your elbows bent 90 degrees and your fingers facing forward.
- Finish the lift by rotating your hands to the ceiling and opening your chest.

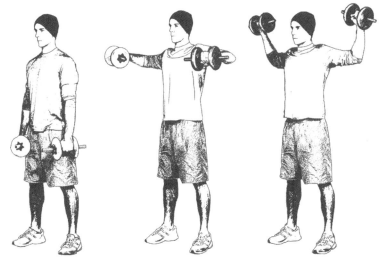

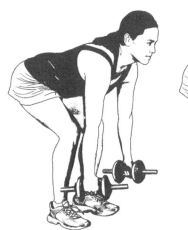 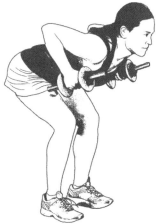

Bent Over Row

- Bend over at your waist, holding two dumbbells lowered toward the floor.
- Lift the weights toward your shoulders.
- Avoid letting your elbows flare too far out to the side.
- Focus on pulling your shoulder blades back and along your spine.

Single Arm Bent Over Row

- Do the same Bent Over Row movement just described, but use a single weight.
- Rest your free arm on your thigh or place it at your waist.

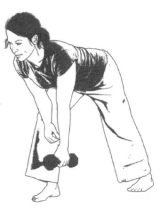 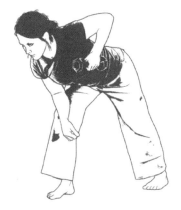

Supported Single Arm Row

- Bend forward at your waist and support yourself on a weight bench with a hand and knee.
- Lift a dumbbell with your free hand towards your chest.
- Focus on pulling your shoulder blade backward.

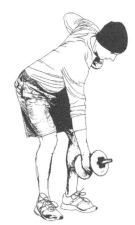

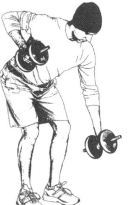

Alternating Row

- Bend forward at your waist as with the Bent Over Row.
- Lift one dumbbell towards your chest while the other dangles toward the floor.
- Alternate the rowing motion from one side to the other.

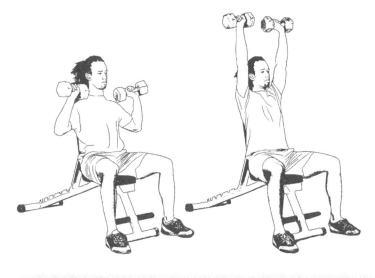

Shoulder Press

- Start in a seated position and lift two dumbbells to shoulder-height.
- Push the weights to the ceiling by straightening your elbows and driving your hands upward.
- Finish by returning your hands to your shoulders.
- Don't let your elbows splay too far out to the side.
- *Variation:* Try this movement standing.

Single Arm Shoulder Press

- Complete the basic Shoulder Press just described, but use one arm rather than two.
- Avoid twisting by keeping your abdominal muscles contracted.

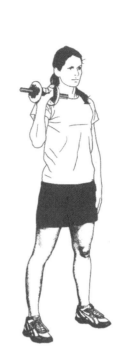
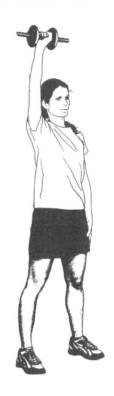

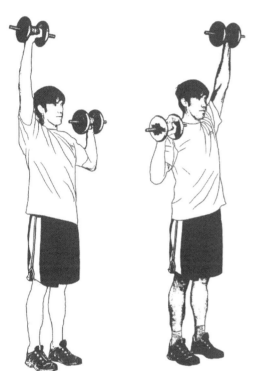

Alternating Shoulder Press

- Use two dumbbells to perform the basic Shoulder Press, but alternate lifting one arm versus the other.
- Stay tight through your trunk and lower body.
- Reach as high as you can on each repetition.

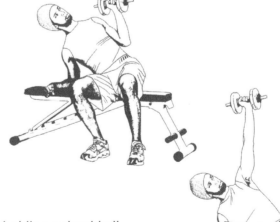

Diagonal Shoulder Press

- Angle your body sideways on a weight bench while holding a dumbbell at your shoulder.
- Straighten your arm, pressing the dumbbell to the ceiling.
- *Variation:* Lie sideways on the ground, or stand with your trunk tipped at an angle.

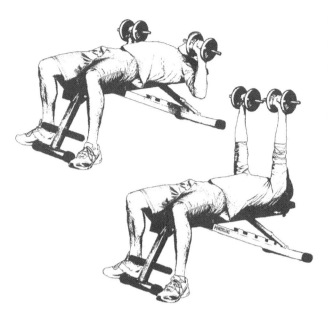

Chest Press

- Lie on your back and hold two dumbbells at your chest.
- Straighten your arms and lift the weights toward the ceiling.
- Try to bring the weights towards each other over your body without crashing them together.

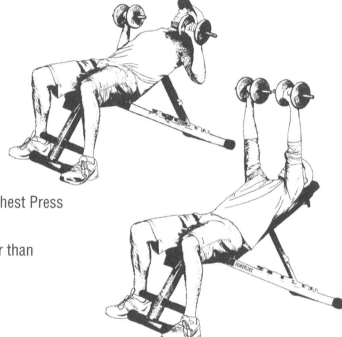

Incline Press

- Use an incline weight bench to perform the basic Chest Press movement.
- Lift your hands straight up toward the ceiling rather than directly over your sternum.

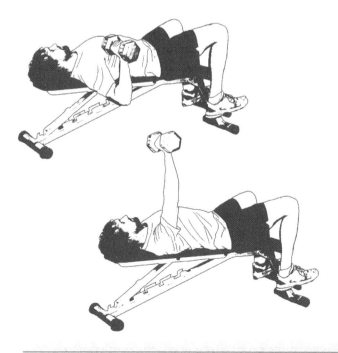

Single Arm Chest Press

- Use one arm to complete a Chest Press.
- Keep your abdominal muscles contracted to prevent trunk rotation.

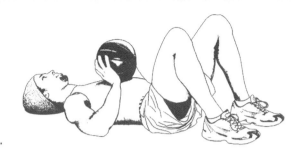

Self Chest Toss

- Lie on your back and hold a medicine ball at your sternum.
- Shoot your hands upward, throwing the ball toward the ceiling.
- Catch the ball and lower it slowly.
- Explode upward again to repeat the movement.

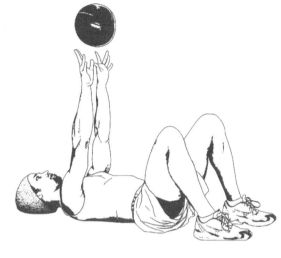

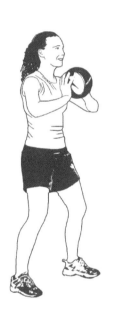

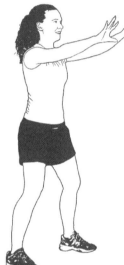

Chest Pass

- Stand with your feet shoulder-width apart while holding a medicine ball at your chest.
- Thrust your hands forward to throw the ball as far forward as you can.

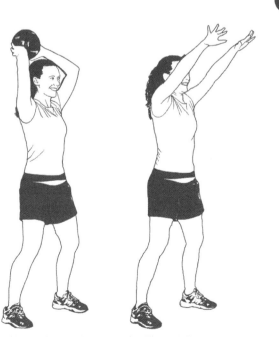

Overhead Pass

- Stand with your feet shoulder-width apart while holding a medicine ball overhead.
- Drive your hands in front of your head as hard as you can to throw the ball forward.
- *Variation:* Do this movement kneeling on the ground.

Chest Fly

- Lie on your back and hold two dumbbells above your chest with your elbows extended.
- Let your arms spread apart, opening your chest.
- Stop when the dumbbells are level with your torso.
- Reverse the motion to bring the dumbbells back above your chest.

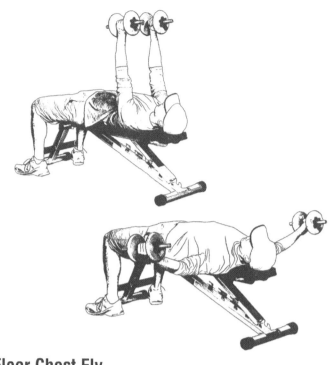

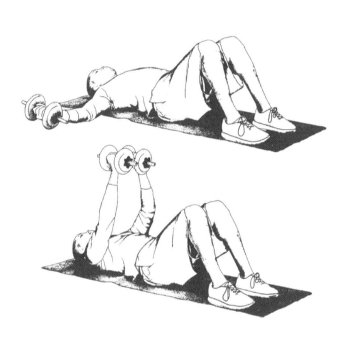

Floor Chest Fly

- Lie on the ground with your knees bent while holding two dumbbells above you.
- Lower the dumbbells to the side, but rest for a moment when they make contact with the floor.
- Return the dumbbells overhead, keeping your arms nearly straight.

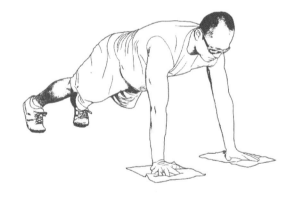

Body-weight Chest Fly

- Get on the ground in a plank position with your hands placed on two wash clothes.
- Spread your arms apart, sliding your hands outward along to floor.
- Stop when your chest is just a few inches from the ground.
- Reverse the motion, sliding your hands back together to the starting position.

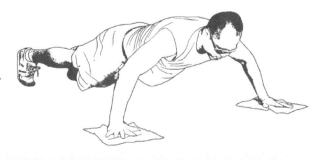

Shoulder Shrug

- Hold two dumbbells by your sides with your shoulders relaxed.
- Tighten your upper back muscles and lift your shoulders to your ears.
- Keep your neck in neutral alignment without letting your head jut forward.

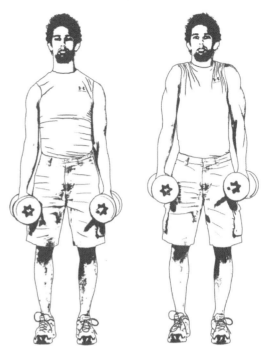

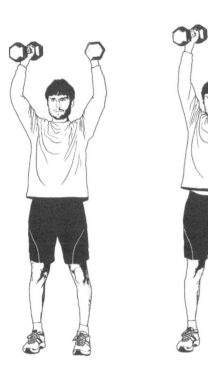

Overhead Shrug

- Hold two dumbbells overhead with your arms extended.
- Shrug your shoulders higher toward your ears.
- Don't let your head protrude forward.

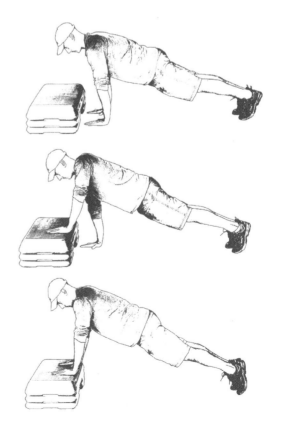

Shoulder Step-up

- Get in a plank position next to a stair.
- Place one hand on the stair, and then walk your second hand up, lifting your body upwards.
- Walk your hands back down from the stair one at a time.
- Alternate which hand leads the step-up movement.

Plate Curl & Raise

- Use two hands to hold a weight plate at your waist.
- Bend your elbows, curling the plate to your chest.
- Finish by lifting the plate over your head.
- *Make it harder:* Press the weight toward the ceiling, fully extending your elbows.

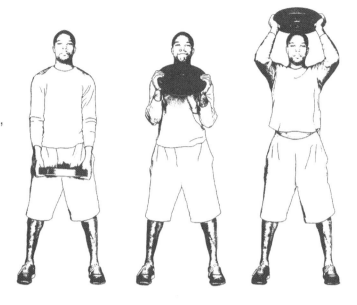

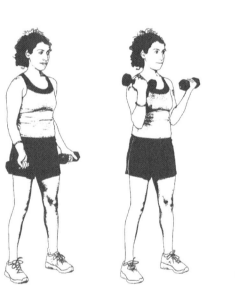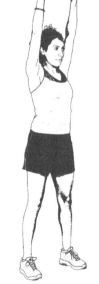

Curl & Press

- Hold two dumbbells by your waist.
- Curl the weights to your shoulders.
- Then perform a Shoulder Press to raise the weights overhead.

Single Arm Curl & Press

- Curl a single dumbbell to your shoulder, and then press it overhead.
- Let your opposite hand rest on your pelvis for extra stability.

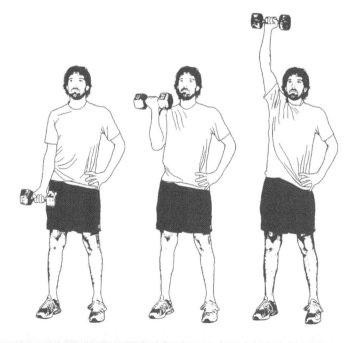

Diagonal Shoulder Raise - Inward

- Hold a single dumbbell out to the side, approximately one foot from your hips.
- Lift the dumbbell inward and across your body, so it ends above your opposite shoulder.
- Reverse direction to return to the starting position.

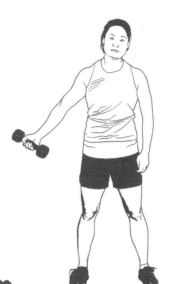
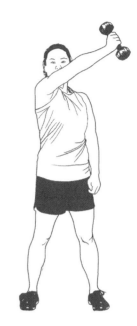

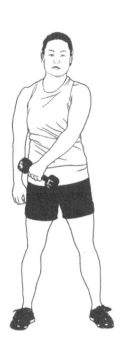
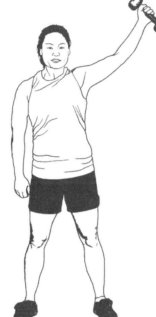

Diagonal Shoulder Raise - Outward

- Start by holding a single dumbbell across your body, near your opposite hip.
- Raise the dumbbell upward and outward, drawing a diagonal across your body.
- Finish with the weight held out to the side on a 45 degree angle.

Chapter 4

"Why is it that athletes and those interested in building serious muscle kneel to the temple of the barbell?"

Barbell Barbarian

Powerlifters and bodybuilders live and die by them. Sports stars swear by them for improved performance. And Arnold Schwarzenegger most definitely used one to bulk up for Conan the Barbarian.

What are we talking about?

Barbells of course!

Why is it that athletes and those interested in building serious muscle kneel to the temple of the barbell?

The answer is plain and simple: They allow you to lift a lot of weight, and with a high degree of stability. Elite powerlifters can squat in excess of 900 lbs and bench press upwards of 650 lbs with a barbell. Attempt either of those lifts with a pair of dumbbells and your arms would probably rip off.

The design of a barbell allows for a nearly endless progression of weight to be added. Thus, it's the tool of choice for when you want to do some serious weight lifting.

In this chapter you'll learn a huge variety of lifts that can be performed with a barbell. With over a dozen squats, multiple lunges, deadlifts, and upper body movements there is certainly enough to keep you from getting bored. There are even a few unconventional core-strengthening exercises thrown in for fun!

One thing that you'll probably notice right away is that single joint (isolation) movements are a rarity in this chapter. There are a few sprinkled here and there, but by and large the barbell is your tool of choice for big, compound skills using multiple joints and muscle groups. May it be your most trusted companion in the pursuit of strength and explosive power!

Without further adieu, I present: The Barbell.

Back Squat

- Hold the barbell behind your shoulders with your elbows tucked in.
- Open your stance and let your knees rotate out.
- Arch your back to maintain the curve of your spine.
- Drop your hips until your thighs are at least parallel with the ground.
- Push the floor, staying tight in your trunk, to return to standing.

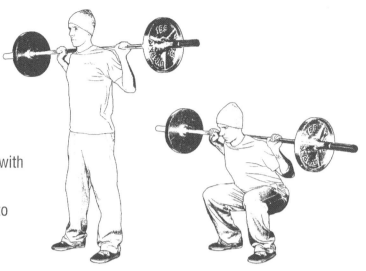

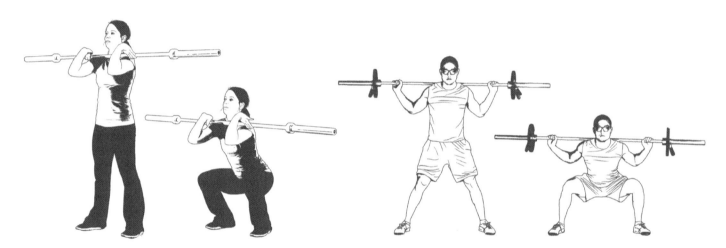

Front Squat

- Hold the barbell across the top of your chest, near your collarbones.
- Raise your elbows to keep the bar in place with your fingertips.
- Maintain your spine alignment by arching your back.
- Lower into a squat as far as you can go without losing your spinal curve.
- Drive down through your feet to straighten back to standing.
- *Variation:* Let your arms cross in front of your body while holding the bar at your chest with your hands.

Wide Leg Squat

- Start with the barbell in the Back Squat position.
- Widen your stance to nearly double shoulder-width with your feet rotated outward.
- Drop to a squat without letting your knees cave inward.
- Return to stand, staying tight through your core and upper body.

Zercher Squat

- Hold a barbell in the crook of your elbows.
- Lower into a squat as far as you can without losing your back curvature.
- Don't let your knees tip inward.
- Return to standing by pushing through your legs, straight to the ceiling.

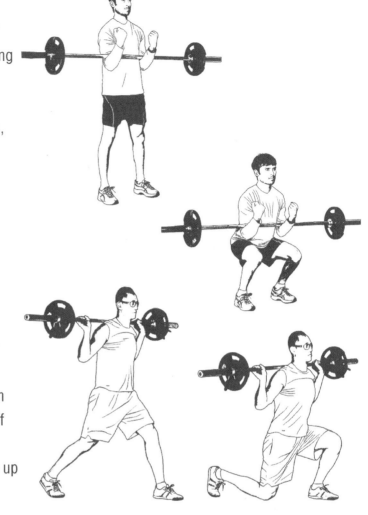

Barbell Split Squat

- Place a barbell across your upper back, and position your feet forward and backward of your trunk.
- Lower into a squat keeping equal weight between your feet, but let the heel of your back leg rise off the ground.
- Try not to shift your weight front or back, but go up and down along a vertical path.

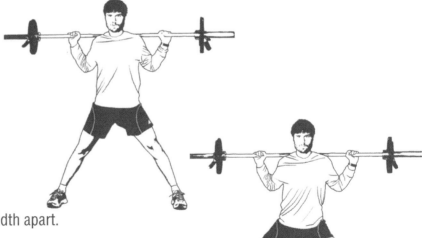

Lateral Split Squat

- Stand with your feet double shoulder-width apart.
- Hold a barbell across your upper back.
- Bend one knee and drop your weight onto the bent leg.
- Keep your other leg straight as you perform a modified single-leg squat.
- Push strong through your flexed leg to return to standing.

Barbell Bulgarian Split Squat

- Hold a barbell across your upper back and shoulders.
- Place one foot behind you on a knee-high bench or box.
- Lower your body straight down, performing a modified single leg squat on your free leg.
- Push the ground with your bottom leg to return to standing.
- Maintain your normal spinal curve throughout the squat.

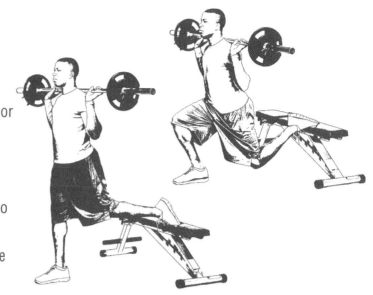

Elevated Front Foot Barbell Split Squat

- Hold a barbell across your upper back and shoulders.
- Pace one foot in front of you, on a small bench or box.
- Lower your body straight down into a split squat position.
- Push the floor through both legs to return to standing.
- Don't let your pelvis tuck under at the bottom of the lift.

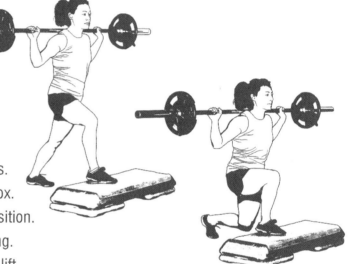

Hack Squat

- Hold a barbell behind your body, near your hips.
- Lower your body straight down into a squat without losing the curve of your spine.
- Don't let your knees drop in or out.
- Push the ground to return to standing.
- *Variation:* Mix-it up with your heels elevated versus flat on the ground.

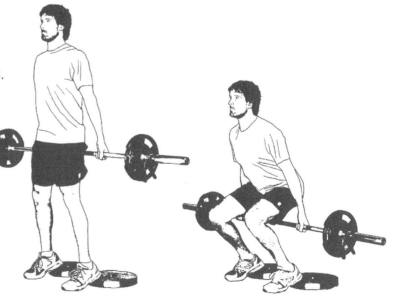

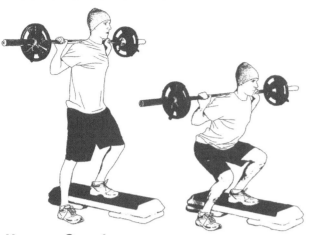

Uneven Squat

- Stand sideways along a stair or small box, holding a barbell across your upper back and shoulders.
- Place one leg on the elevated surface with your toes nearly forward.
- Lower into a modified single leg squat with the majority of your weight on the leg that is on the floor.
- Watch your knee alignment and maintain your spine curve while lowering and returning to stand.

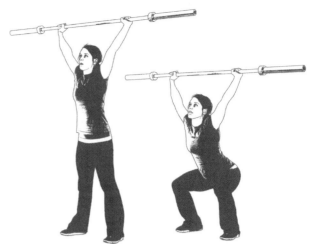

Barbell Overhead Squat

- Hold a barbell overhead with your hands spread in a wide grip.
- Engage your back muscles to pull your shoulder blades down and together.
- Drop into a squat until your thighs are parallel with the floor, or lower if possible.
- Keep the bar overhead and return to standing.

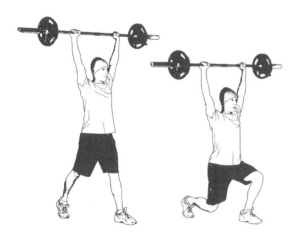

Overhead Split Squat

- Hold a barbell overhead and spread your feet forward and backward in a Split Squat stance.
- Be active in your back and shoulders to keep the barbell directly overhead.
- Lower into a split squat, allowing the heel of your back foot to come up, as you drop your knee down.
- Keep the weight even between your feet, as you return to standing.

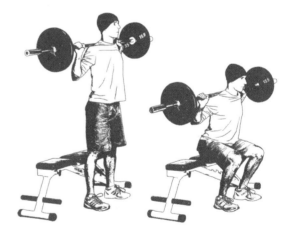

Box/Bench Squat

- Stand in front of a weight bench or plyo box with a barbell in the Back Squat position.
- Lower into a squat and come to rest on the bench or box.
- Maintain your spine curve through out the movement.
- Lift off the seat and return to standing.

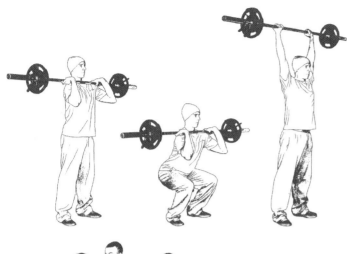

Thruster

- Hold a barbell near your chest, in the Front Squat position.
- Lower into a squat until your thighs are parallel to the floor.
- Explode to a standing position while pressing the barbell overhead.
- Lower the barbell to your chest as you drop back into your squat.

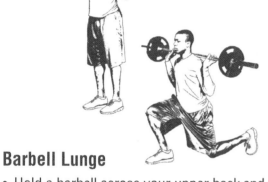

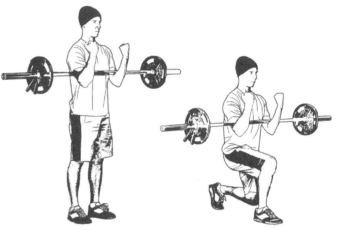

Barbell Lunge

- Hold a barbell across your upper back and shoulders.
- Take a big step forward and shift your weight onto the front leg.
- Keep your knee directly over your foot (don't let it drop in or out).
- Push the ground forcefully with your front leg to return to the starting position.

Zercher Lunge

- Hold a barbell across the front of your body in the crook of your elbows.
- Take a big step forward and shift your weight onto the front leg.
- Push the ground forcefully with your front leg to return to the starting position.

Barbell Side Lunge

- Hold a barbell across your upper back and shoulders.
- Take a large step to the side and shift your weight onto that leg.
- Watch your knee alignment. Don't let it drop in or out too much.
- Push the ground with your outside leg to step back to the starting position.

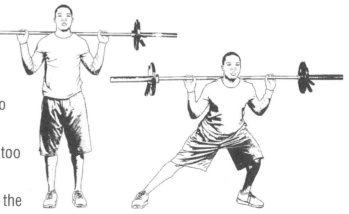

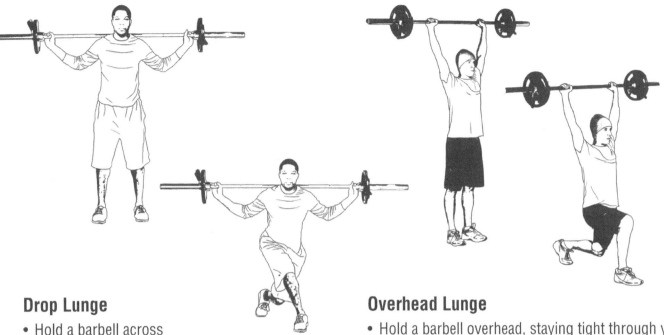

Drop Lunge

- Hold a barbell across
  your upper back and shoulders.
- Take a step backward and behind the front leg.
- Lower your body into crouched position.
- Push off from your back leg and stay tight through
  your front leg to return to the starting position
- Imagine pushing your front leg out to the side as
  you stand up.

Overhead Lunge

- Hold a barbell overhead, staying tight through your
  upper back and shoulders.
- Take a large step forward and shift your weight to
  the front leg.
- Let your front knee bend until it is over the foot,
  and then push backward to return to the starting
  position.

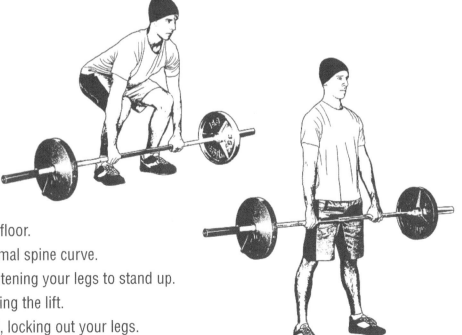

Deadlift

- Stand with your feet
  shoulder-width apart.
- Bend your hips and knees so that
  you can grasp the barbell from the floor.
- Keep your back arched with its normal spine curve.
- Tighten your grip and begin straightening your legs to stand up.
- Keep the bar close to your legs during the lift.
- Finish by driving your hips forward, locking out your legs.

Barbell Sumo Deadlift

- Spread your legs nearly double shoulder-width apart.
- Let your feet rotate outward.
- Lower your body to grasp the barbell from the floor.
- Arch your back to maintain your spine position.
- Push the ground to straighten your legs and raise the barbell to your thighs.

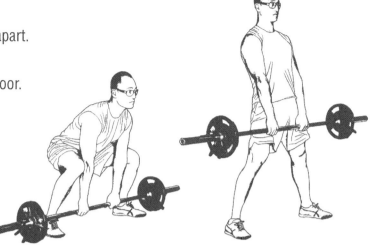

Stiff Leg Deadlift

- Stand with your feet shoulder-width apart.
- Bend forward from your waist, hinging through your hips.
- Bend your knees slightly to maintain your spine in a slight arch.
- Grasp the barbell and lift upward, keeping it near your legs.
- Push your hips forward to finish the lift.

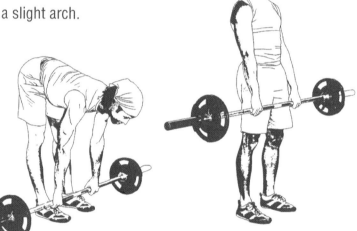

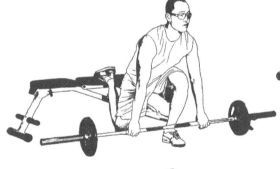

Bulgarian Split Deadlift

- Place one foot behind you on a knee-high bench or box.
- Bend forward to grab a barbell from the floor.
- Straighten your bottom leg to raise yourself to a standing position.
- Keep the barbell close to your leg.
- Drive your hips forward at the top of the lift.

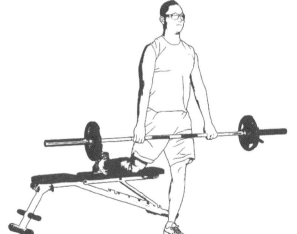

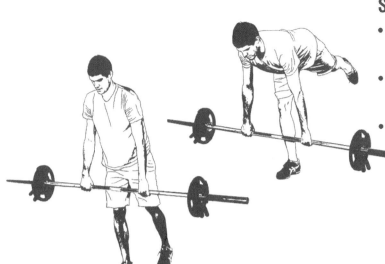

Single Leg Deadlift

- Balance on one leg and bend forward from your hips to grab a barbell from the floor.
- Raise your chest and lift the barbell up to your thighs.
- Arch your back to maintain your spinal curve.

Barbell Good Morning

- Stand with your feet shoulder-width apart, holding a barbell across your upper back and shoulders.
- Hinge forward through your hips, dropping your chest and pushing your butt backward.
- Arch your back to maintain your spinal curve.
- Tighten your legs and back, and then drive your hips forward to lift your chest up to the starting position.

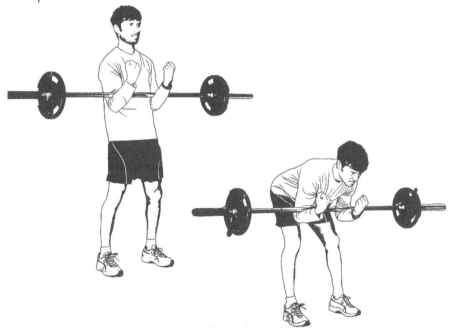

Zercher Good Morning

- Hold a barbell in the crook of your elbows.
- Hinge forward through your hips, dropping your chest and pushing your butt backward.
- Stop when you can't go any lower without losing your spinal curve.
- Tighten your legs and back, and then drive your hips forward to return to the starting position.

Split Good Morning

- Place one foot in front of you, elevated on weight plates if possible.
- Hold a barbell across your upper back and shoulders.
- Hinge forward through your hips, dropping your shoulders and pushing your butt backward.
- Return to standing by driving your hips forward and lifting your chest.

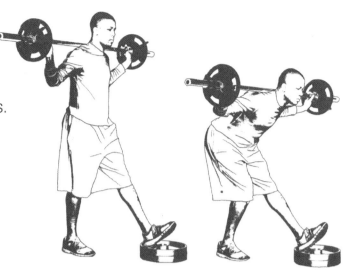

Seated Good Morning

- Sit on a bench or box in a straddle position.
- Hold a barbell across your upper back and shoulder.
- Hinge forward from your hips, bringing your chest to the bench.
- Tighten your back muscles and lift your trunk to the upright position.

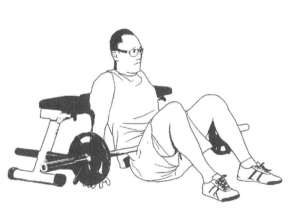

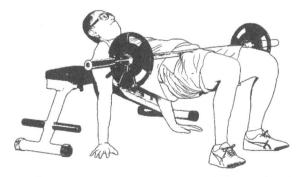

Barbell Hip Thrust

- Sit on the floor with your back against a bench or box.
- Place a barbell across your lower pelvis, near your thighs.
- Tighten your legs and drive your hips upward.
- *Variation:* Try it with your arms across your chest.

Barbell Calf Raise

- Hold a barbell across your upper back and shoulders.
- Stand with your feet shoulder-width apart.
- Tighten your calves and rise upward onto your tiptoes.
- Go as high as you can, and then lower slowly.

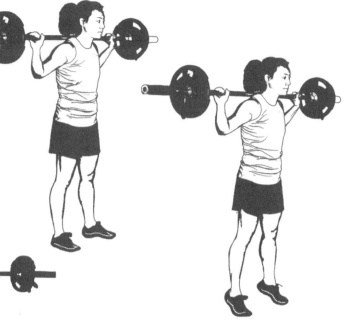

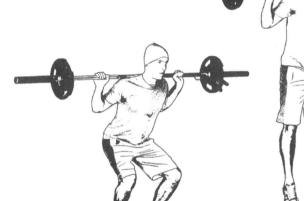

Barbell Squat Jump

- Place a barbell across your shoulders in the Back Squat position.
- Lower to a partial squat and then explode off the ground into a jump.
- Land softly, absorbing the momentum with your legs.

Hang Clean

- Stand with your feet shoulder-width apart.
- Bend forward and hold a barbell at your lower thighs.
- Tighten your back and legs, and then drive your hips forward explosively.
- Simultaneously stand tall while pulling the barbell to your shoulders.
- Do not try to curl the barbell; it should come up in one smooth motion.

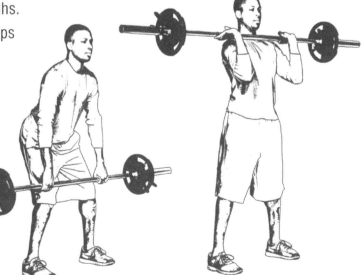

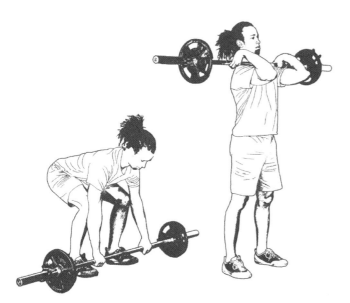

Power Clean

- Bend forward at your hips to grasp a barbell from the floor.
- Arch your back to maintain your natural spine curve.
- Explode upward to a standing position while pulling the barbell to your shoulders.
- Lift your elbows at the top of the movement.
- *Variation:* Drop into a squat while bringing the bar to your shoulders, and then stand up (aka "Squat Clean").

Clean & Press

- Perform the same initial movements as a Power Clean.
- Once you have the barbell to your shoulders, press it overhead.
- Finish by locking your hips and driving your head and chest forward.

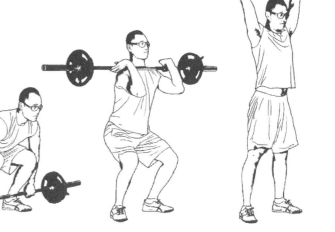

Snatch

- Bend forward to grasp a barbell from the floor.
- Arch your back to maintain your spinal curve.
- Drop into a squat while pulling the barbell up and overhead in one smooth and explosive motion.
- Rise to a standing position once the barbell is locked overhead.

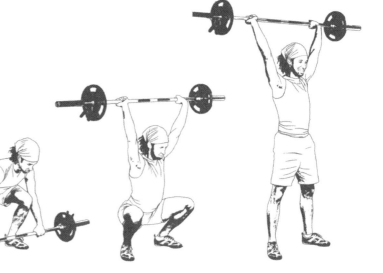

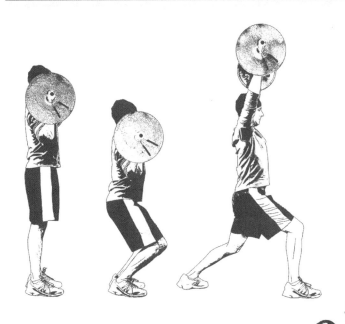

Split Jerk

- Hold a barbell across the front of your shoulders.
- Drop to a slight squat, and then explode upward and lunge one foot forward and one foot backward.
- Simultaneously press the bar overhead and drive your chest forward.
- Bring your feet back together and stand tall with the bar overhead.

Push Press

- Hold a barbell across the front of your shoulders.
- Drop to a slight squat then explode upward, thrusting the barbell overhead.
- Finish by locking out your arms and bringing your head and chest forward.

Barbell Burpee

- Get in a push-up position on the ground with your hands placed on a barbell.
- Jump up to a squat while bringing the barbell to your shoulders.
- Stand up and press the barbell to the ceiling.

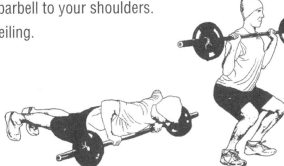

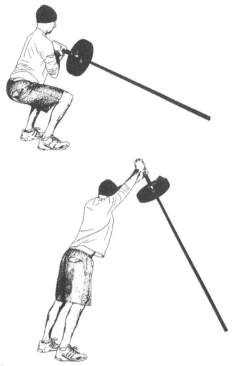

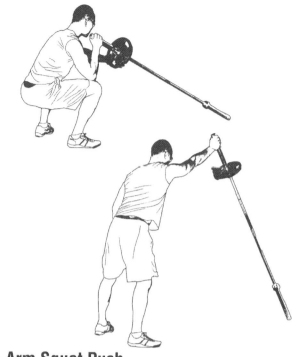

Squat Push

- Take weights off one end of a barbell and tuck that end into a corner or somewhere that it won't slip.
- Hold the weighted end of the barbell with both hands at your chest.
- Drop to a squat.
- Explode into a standing position while pushing the barbell up and away from you.

Single Arm Squat Push

- Perform the same basic motion as the Squat Push, but use a single arm.
- Try to keep your elbow tucked in to your side.
- Finish the movement by fully extending your arm and hips.

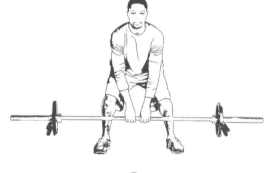

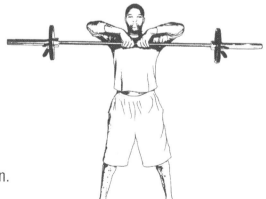

Sumo Deadlift High Pull

- Assume the Sumo Deadlift starting position.
- Use a narrow grip to lift the barbell from the floor.
- Tighten your legs to start standing up.
- Quickly pull the barbell upward in a fast motion.
- Finish with your hips locked and your hands near your chin.

Barbell Bent Over Row

- Bend over and hold a barbell in front of your knees.
- Arch your back to maintain your spine curve.
- Pull the barbell to your chest.
- Lower it slowly back to the starting position.

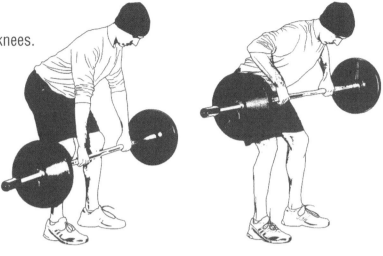

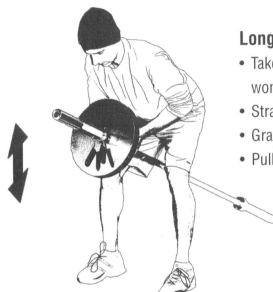

Long Bar Row

- Take weight off one end of a barbell and tuck it into a corner so it won't slide.
- Straddle the barbell and get into a bent-over position.
- Grasp the weighted end of the barbell beneath the weight plate.
- Pull the barbell to your chest.

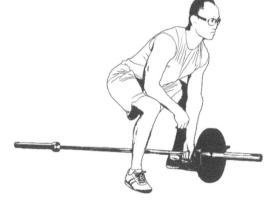

Single Arm Long Bar Row

- Begin in the Long Bar Row position.
- Hold the weighted end with one arm.
- Position your free arm on your thigh for support.
- Pull the barbell to your chest with one arm.

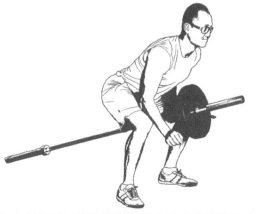

Upright Row

- Stand with your feet spread shoulder-width apart.
- Hold a barbell at your thighs with a medium-narrow grip.
- Pull the barbell to your chin in one smooth motion.

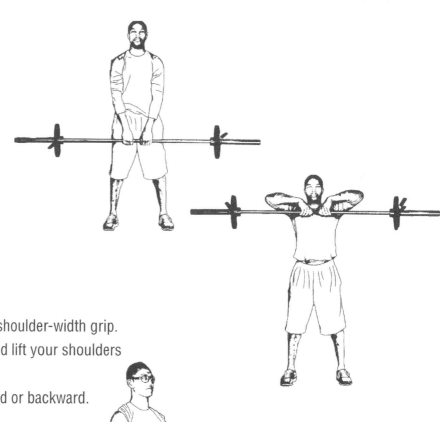

Barbell Shrug

- Hold a barbell at your thighs with a shoulder-width grip.
- Tighten your upper back muscles and lift your shoulders to your ears.
- Don't let your shoulders rock forward or backward.
- Lower the bar back to your thighs.

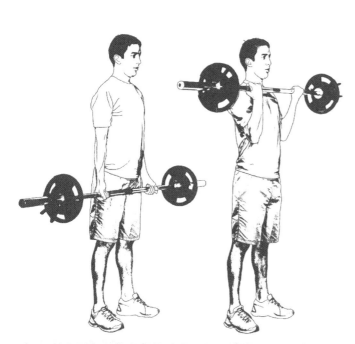

Barbell Bicep Curl

- Hold a barbell at your thighs with your palms facing forward.
- Tighten your biceps to lift the barbell to your collarbones.
- Try not to rock and forth; isolate the movement to your elbows.
- Lower the weight slowly to the starting position.

Barbell Wrist Curl (Behind the Back)

• Hold a barbell behind your back with your palms facing away from you.

• Tighten your forearms to curl your wrists upward.

• Raise your knuckles as high as you can, and then reverse directions.

• *Variation:* Try a wrist curl in front of your body with your palms facing forward.

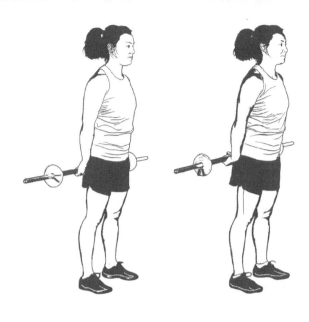

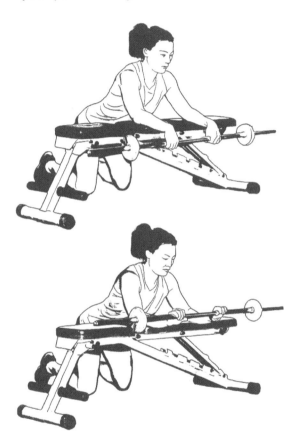

Barbell Reverse Wrist Curl

• Kneel on the floor with your forearms supported on a bench.

• Hold a barbell with your palms facing the floor.

• Tighten your forearms to extend your wrists and lift the barbell upward.

• Isolate the movement to your wrists, and go as high as you can before reversing directions.

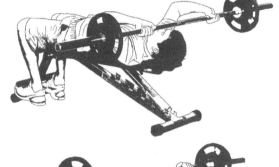

Barbell Tricep Extension

• Lie on a bench and hold a barbell over your chest with your arms extended.

• Allow your elbows to bend and lower the weight above your head.

• Keep your elbows pointed to the ceiling.

• Extend your elbows and raise the barbell back over your chest.

• *Variation:* Try the movement while lying on the floor.

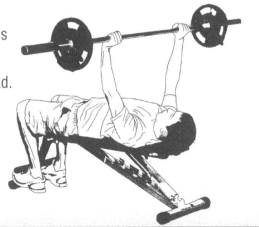

Bench Press

- Lie on a bench and hold a barbell over your chest.
- Lower the barbell your chest.
- Tighten your trunk and lower body while pressing your feet into the floor.
- Push the barbell back to the ceiling.

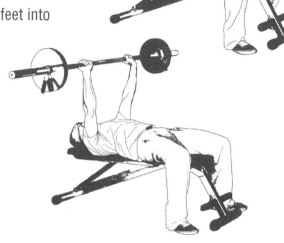

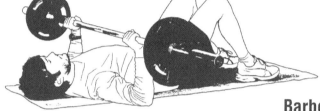

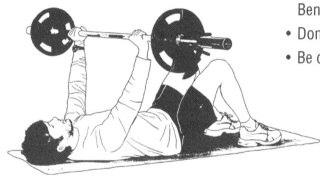

Barbell Floor Press

- Lie on the floor and perform the same basic motion as the Bench Press.
- Don't let your pelvis rise into the air.
- Be careful not to slam your elbows onto the ground.

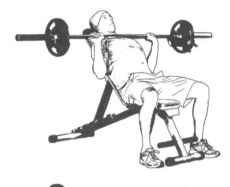

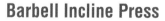

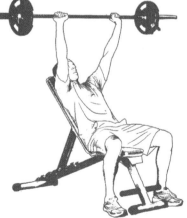

Barbell Incline Press

- Sit in an incline bench with a barbell across your upper chest.
- Press the barbell to the ceiling and then return it to your sternum.
- Don't let your elbows flare out to the side during the up and down motion.

Neider Press

- Stand with your feet shoulder-width apart.
- Raise a barbell to your chest.
- Press the barbell away from you until your arms are fully extended.
- Pull the barbell back to your chest.

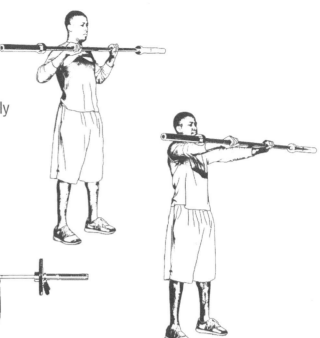

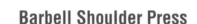

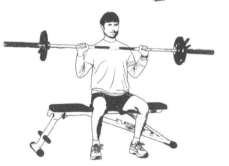

Barbell Shoulder Press

- Stand with your feet shoulder-width apart.
- Hold a barbell across the front of your shoulders and upper chest.
- Push the barbell to the ceiling.
- Don't let your elbows rotate out too far.
- Lower the barbell back to your chest.

Seated Barbell Shoulder Press

- Sit on a bench or box and perform a Shoulder Press.
- Keep your trunk muscles tight and limit any spine motion.
- Raise the barbell fully overhead and lock your arms before lowering.

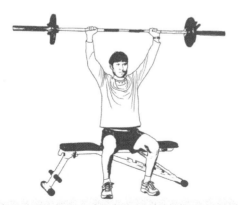

Sots Press

- Assume a deep squat with a barbell across your upper chest in the Front Squat Position.
- Press the barbell to the ceiling, fully locking your arms out overhead.
- Return the barbell to the starting position while still in the deep squat.

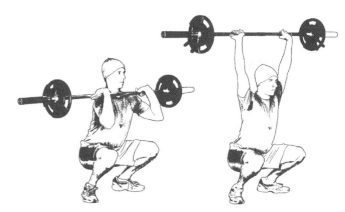

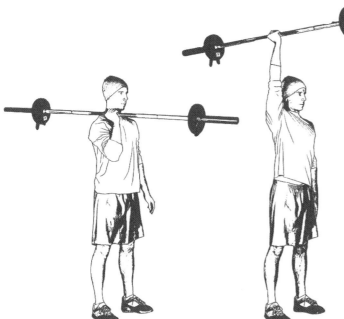

Javelin Press

- Hold a barbell at your shoulder with one hand, as if you were about to throw a javelin.
- Press the barbell to the ceiling, fully extending your elbow and pulling your shoulder blade down your back.
- Minimize excess sway in the barbell, by using active wrist control.

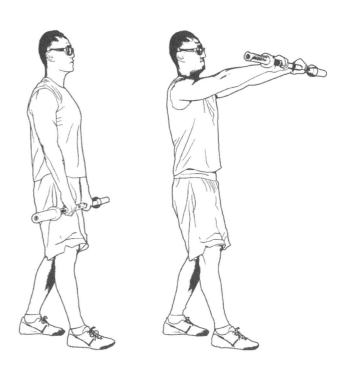

Barbell Forward Raise

- Stand with your feet staggered 8 to 12 inches apart.
- Hold a barbell across your upper thighs.
- Tighten your upper back muscles and lift the barbell to chest-level.
- Keep your arms straight during the motion and lower the barbell slowly.

Barbell Overhead Raise

- Stand with your feet staggered or in shoulder-width position.
- Hold a barbell across your upper thighs.
- Tighten your upper back muscles and start lifting the barbell upward.
- Keep your arms straight and lift the barbell overhead in an arcing motion.
- Lower it back down in a smooth arc.

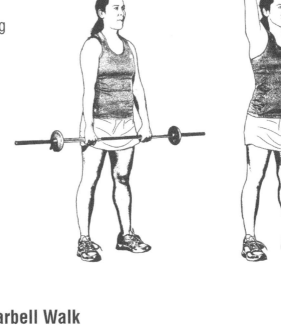

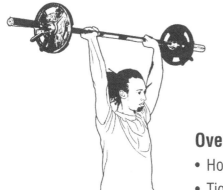

Overhead Barbell Walk

- Hold a barbell overhead with your arms fully extended.
- Tighten your abdominal muscles and begin walking forward.
- Keep the barbell overhead as you walk across the floor.

Barbell Roll-out

- Get in a kneeling position, grasping a barbell in front of you on the ground.
- Tighten your abdominal muscles and push the barbell away from you.
- Let your trunk lower to the ground as the barbell rolls forward.
- Reverse directions when you are almost fully elongated.

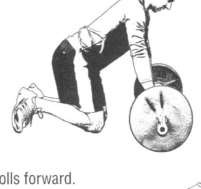

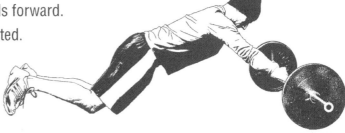

Barbell Roll-out (Standing)

- Stand with your feet shoulder-width apart and bent forward at the waist.
- Place your hands on a barbell, resting on the ground.
- Tighten your abdominal muscles and push the barbell away from you.
- Let your body lower to the ground as the barbell rolls forward.
- Pull the barbell back toward you to return to the starting position.

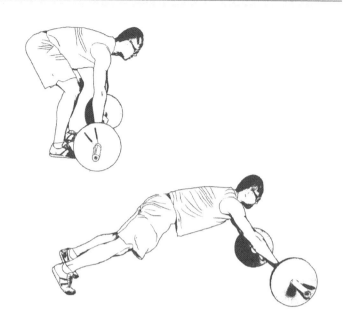

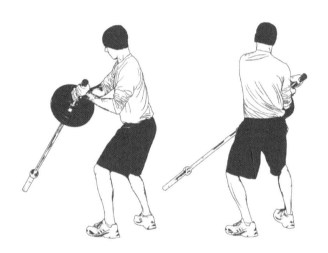

Half Moon

- Take the weight plates off one end of a barbell.
- Tuck the free end of the barbell against a wall and hold the weighted end.
- Drop to a partial squat, twist your trunk and lower the barbell to one side of your body.
- Stand up and perform the same motion on the opposite side.

Barbell Side Bend

- Hold a barbell across your upper back and shoulders.
- Tighten your abdominal muscles and tip one end of the barbell to the floor.
- Stay strong through your trunk and bring the barbell back to the middle.
- Repeat the motion to the opposite side.

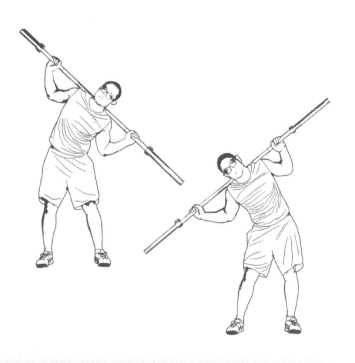

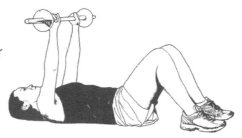

Barbell Sit-up

- Lie on the floor with your knees bent and hold a barbell over your chest.
- Press the barbell to the ceiling as you perform a sit-up.
- Keep your arms fully extended throughout the movement.

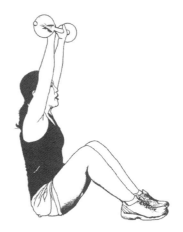

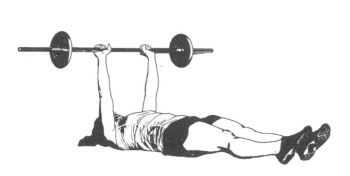

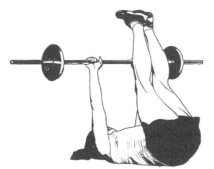

Barbell Hold Leg Raise

- Lie on the floor with your legs extended and hold a barbell over your chest.
- Tighten your abdominal muscles and lift your legs toward the barbell.
- Keep your arms fully extended through out the movement.
- Lower your legs slowly without letting your back arch.

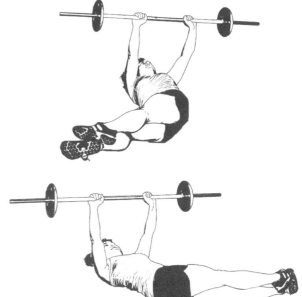

Barbell Windshield Wipers

- Lie on the floor and hold a barbell over your chest.
- Raise your legs to 90 degrees off the ground.
- Tighten your abdominal muscles and allow your legs to lower to one side of your body.
- Raise your legs back to vertical and then lower them to the other side.

Chapter 5

"The mass of a kettlebell is offset from the handle, which forces you to use extra stabilizing muscles to control its motion during a lift."

Killer KBs

Unless you just woke up from a 10-year coma, you've probably already seen kettlebells in a weight room, on late-night TV, or down the fitness aisle of your local box store. These Russian strength tools are best described as "cannonballs with handles," and are basically a sphere of cast iron with a grip, looped over the top. They come in a variety of weights and sizes and have taken the fitness world by storm.

What makes a kettlebell such a killer piece of workout equipment?

- **Versatility:** Aside from allowing you to perform almost all of the movements that you can do with dumbbell, you can also swap a kettlebell for many medicine ball and weight plate exercises.

- **Stability:** The mass of a kettlebell is offset from the handle, which forces you to use extra stabilizing muscles to control its motion during a lift.

- **Grip:** The unique shape of the handle makes it easy to do a variety of exercise movements that would be difficult (if not dangerous) with a dumbbell. Try passing a 50 lb dumbbell between your legs from one hand to the other — it's way too awkward!

- **Cardio:** Sub-maximal high repetition lifts with a kettlebell, such as a swing or snatch, are an effective method of getting a cardiovascular burn. Plus, they are way more engaging then slogging away on a dreadmill.

If you're just getting started outfitting your own home gym, I'd recommend getting at least two kettlebells: One that you can lift for upwards of 20 to 30 repetitions for swings, et cetera, and then another that is 10 to 20 pounds heavier for more serious weight lifting.

Prior to digging into the skills, let's go over a definition of the *rack position*. This refers to a common way of holding the kettlebell, by the handle near your shoulder. It is a very stable position and allows for many progressions. The weight should be resting on the outside of your wrist, with your elbow tucked into your ribs and your wrist held in a neutral position.

Enjoy the 40+ movements in this chapter, but be forewarned: They are highly addictive!

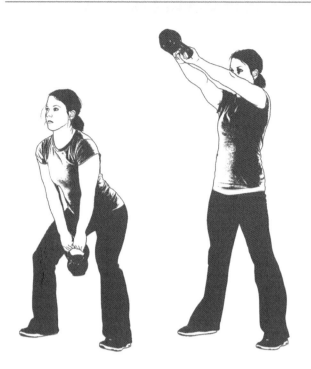

Kettlebell Swing

- Begin in a semi-squat with your feet greater than shoulder-width apart.
- Swing the kettlebell upward with both hands, pushing forcefully through your feet and driving your hips forward.
- Stop when the weight is almost overhead, then lower to the starting position.
- Keep your arms nearly straight through out the swing.

Single Arm Kettlebell Swing

- Perform the same basic motion as the Kettlebell Swing, but use one hand instead of two.
- Try to keep the weight centered near the midline of your body.
- Be cautious to avoid hitting your leg on either the up or down swing.

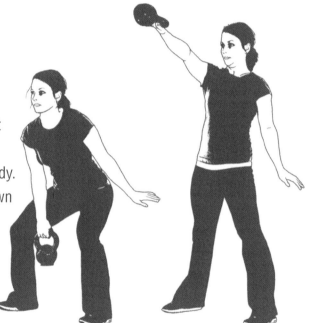

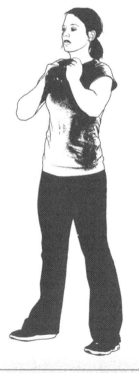

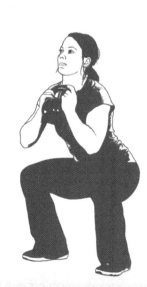

Kettlebell Squat

- Center a kettlebell at your chest, using two hands to grasp the handle.
- Perform a full-depth squat, dropping as far as you can without reversing your lumbar curve.
- Stay active through your feet with your weight even from your heels to your toes.

Single Kettlebell Front Squat

- Hold a single kettlebell in the rack position over your shoulder.
- Keep your elbow raised as you complete a full-depth squat.
- Stay active through your trunk and core muscles to avoid rotation.

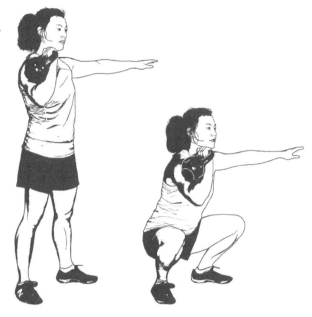

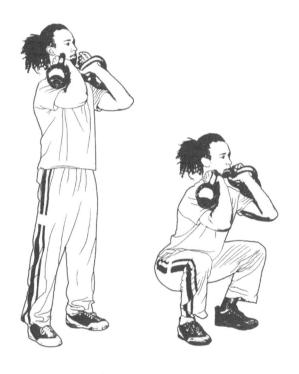

Kettlebell Front Squat

- Hold two kettlebells in the rack position over your shoulders.
- Drop down to a squat while lifting actively through your elbows.
- *Make it harder*: Use kettlebells of different weights for an asymmetrical challenge.

Kettlebell Split Squat

- Stand with one foot in front of the other, keeping your weight spread evenly between your legs.
- Hold two kettlebells on both sides of your body, near your thighs.
- Lower to the floor into a split squat, bending both knees.
- *Variation:* Try elevating either your front or back leg on a small stair or box.

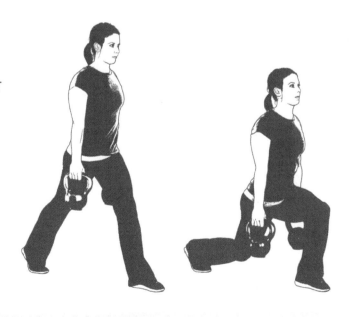

Kettlebell Tiptoe Squat

- Hold one or two kettlebells near your chest in the rack position.
- Drop into a deep squat, letting your heels come off the ground.
- Try to stay balanced on your tiptoes as you raise and lower again.

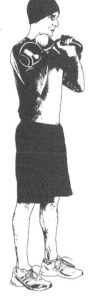
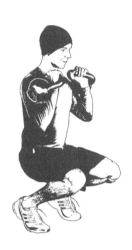

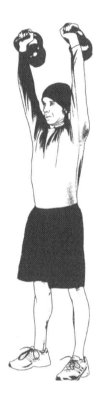
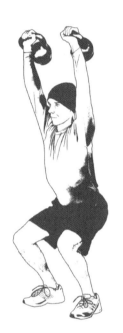

Kettlebell Overhead Squat

- Hold two kettlebells overhead, with your arms extended and shoulders pulled back.
- Lower into a squat as deep as you can, without losing your balance or the curve of your lumbar spine.
- Keep your arms overhead during the entire movement.

Kettlebell Deadlift

- Place your feet on either side of a kettlebell resting on the floor.
- Bend your knees and hips so that you can grasp the handle with both hands.
- Keep your spine slightly arched and chest lifted.
- Straighten your knees and drive your hips forward to stand and lift the weight from the floor.

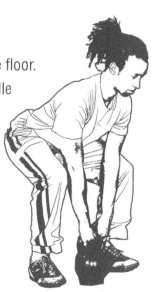
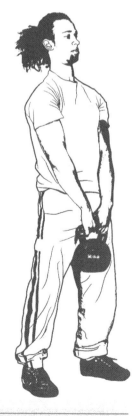

Kettlebell Suitcase Deadlift

- Use one hand to grasp the handle of a kettlebell resting on the outside of one leg.
- Move through a basic deadlift, keeping the weight on the outside of your leg and your arm straight.
- Don't reverse your lumbar curvature.

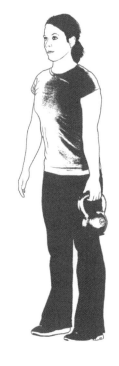
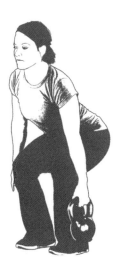

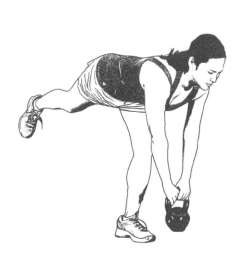
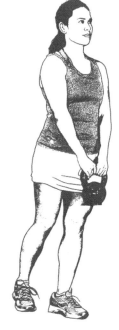

Kettlebell Single Leg Deadlift

- Balance on one leg, using two hands to grasp the handle of a kettlebell in front of your body.
- Hinge forward at your waist to raise and lower the weight from the floor.
- Try to keep your back and knee as straight as possible.

Kettlebell Pistol Squat

- Raise one leg in front of your body, and hold a kettlebell at your chest with two hands.
- Keep the elevated foot off the floor and lower into a single leg squat.
- If necessary, extend the kettlebell forward as a counter-weight for balance.

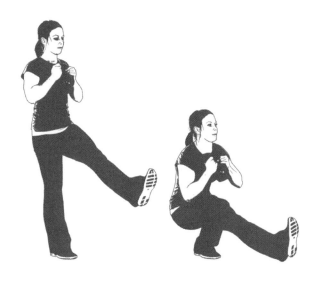

Kettlebell Reverse Lunge

- Hold a kettlebell at your chest with two hands.
- Thrust one leg behind you and lower into a reverse lunge.
- Return to standing by extending your front leg and pushing off your back leg.
- *Variation:* Switch legs on every repetition or do multiple lunges on one side.

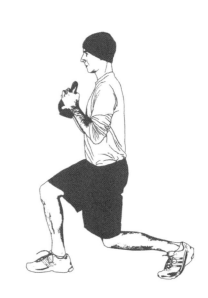

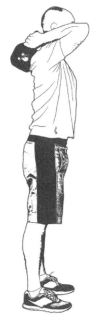
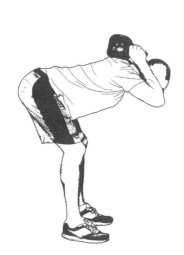

Kettlebell Good Morning

- Hold a kettlebell between your upper shoulders, using two hands.
- Hinge forward at your waist, in a bowing motion.
- Keep your back straight, but allow a slight bend at your knees.
- Drive your hips forward to lift yourself back to a standing position.

Kneeling Get-up

- Start on the ground in a kneeling position, holding a kettlebell at your chest.
- Place one foot forward, and then lift yourself to a standing position.
- Reverse the motion to return to kneeling.

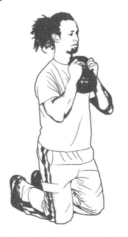
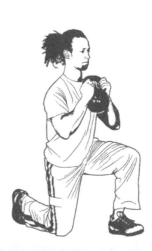
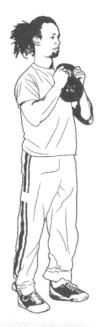

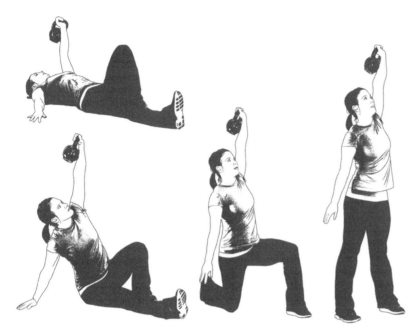

Turkish Get-up

- Lie on the ground, holding a kettlebell by your shoulder.
- Extend the weight to the ceiling, while bending your knee on the same side.
- Use your opposite hand to prop yourself into a sitting position.
- Place the extended leg behind you, so you are now half-kneeling.
- Stand up on your front leg, keeping the kettlebell raised to the ceiling the whole time.
- Reverse the sequence to return to the floor.

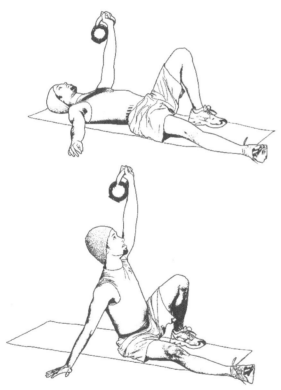

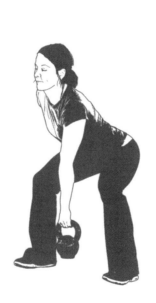

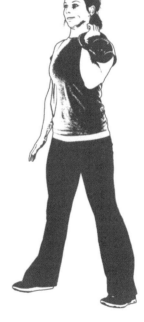

Get-up Sit-up

- Perform the first half of a Turkish Get-up, keeping a kettlebell overhead the entire time.
- Rise to the sitting position and then return to the floor.
- Minimize how hard you use the opposite arm so that you emphasize abdominal strength.

Kettlebell Clean

- Bend forward to grab a single kettlebell positioned in front of you on the floor.
- Extend your legs and drive your hips forward, as you lift the weight from the ground.
- Raise the kettlebell upward so that it comes to rest near your shoulder, in the rack position.

Kettlebell Snatch

- Start in the same beginning position as the Kettlebell Clean.
- Explode upward in a standing motion, while you lift the weight directly overhead.
- Lock your arm overhead as you finish straightening your knees and hips.
- *Variation:* Try lifting the weight overhead in a swinging motion versus a pulling motion.

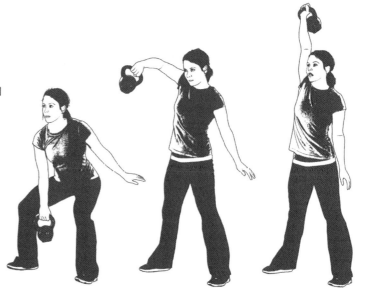

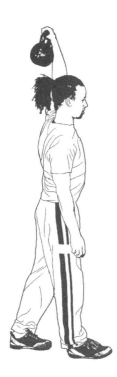

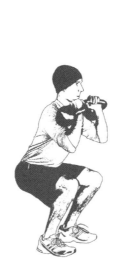

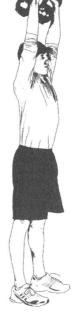

Waiter Carry

- Raise a single kettlebell overhead, with your elbow locked out and shoulder blade pulled backward.
- Stay tight through your trunk as you walk back and forth, holding the weight overhead.

Kettlebell Thruster

- Hold two kettlebells at your shoulders in the rack position.
- Drop to a squat, and then explode upward to stand, while you push the weights to the ceiling.
- Finish with your arms and knees locked out, then drop back to a squat and repeat.

Windmill

- Stand with your feet shoulder-width apart, with one foot rotated outward 90 degrees.
- Raise a kettlebell overhead on the side of your foot that is facing forward.
- Bend over at your waist so that you can touch your free hand to the foot that is rotated outward.
- Hold the kettlebell to the ceiling the entire time.
- Return to standing.

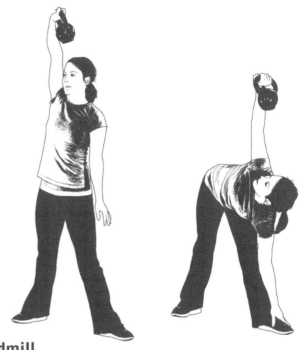

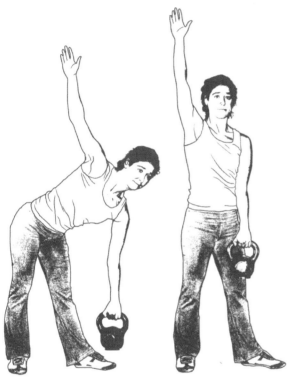

Low Windmill

- Start with your feet in the same basic position as the Windmill.
- Hold a kettlebell in one hand near the thigh of the foot that is rotated outward.
- Raise your other hand overhead.
- Hinge at your waist to lower the kettlebell toward the floor.
- Stay tight through your trunk, to protect your spinal alignment.
- Return to standing.

Double Windmill

- Perform the basic motion of a Kettlebell Windmill, but hold a second kettlebell in your free hand.
- Keep your trunk and abdominal muscles engaged throughout the movement.

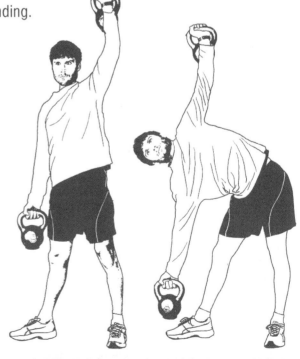

Kettlebell Arm Bar

- Lie on the floor as if you were going to do a Turkish Get-up, with a kettlebell overhead and one leg bent.
- Roll onto your free side, but keep the weight lifted to the ceiling.
- Retract your shoulder blade while keeping the weight extended above you.

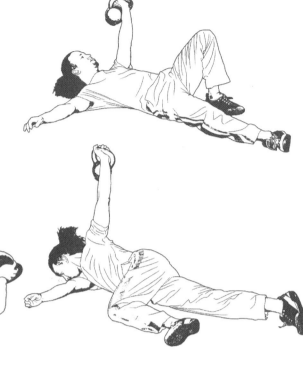

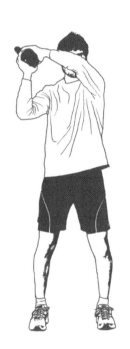 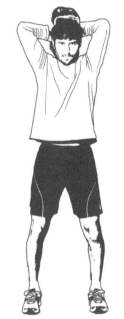 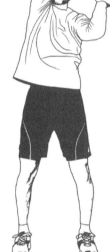 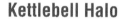

Kettlebell Halo

- Hold a kettlebell with two hands, keeping it level with your head.
- Rotate the weight around your head in a circular motion.

Kettlebell Waist Circles

- Grasp the handle of a kettlebell with one hand, and begin moving it behind your back.
- Reach backward with your free hand to grab the weight.
- Switch hands and keep the weight moving around your waist in a circular motion.

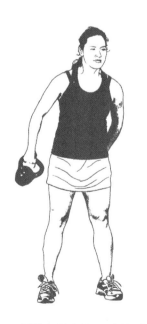 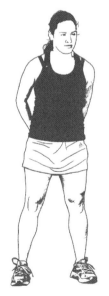 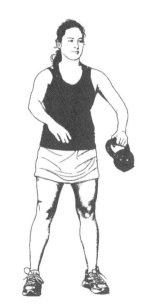

Kettlebell Figure Eights

- Get in a semi-squat with your legs spread nearly double shoulder-width.
- Hold a kettlebell with a single hand, and swing it between your knees.
- Grab the handle with your free hand, from the opposite side of your body.
- Move the weight through your knees in a figure eight motion.

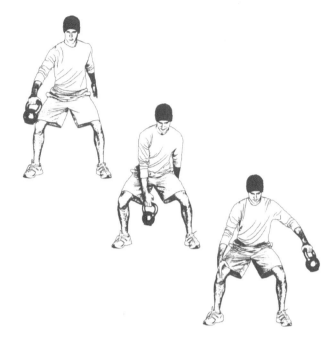

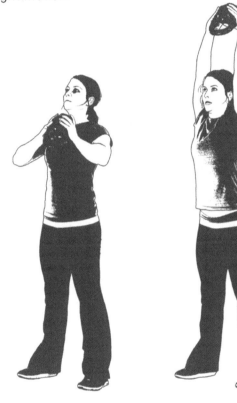

Kettlebell Overhead Press

- Use two hands to hold a kettlebell near your sternum.
- Press the weight overhead.
- Lock out your elbows, and then return to the starting position.

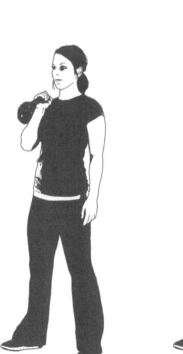
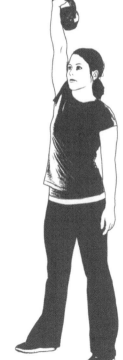

Kettlebell Shoulder Press

- Hold a single kettlebell near one shoulder, in the rack position.
- Drive the weight overhead in a basic Shoulder Press motion.

Kettlebell Push Press

- Start with a kettlebell at your shoulder, in the rack position.
- Drop to a quarter squat, then explode upward, pressing the weight to the ceiling.
- Lower it to your shoulder, and repeat.

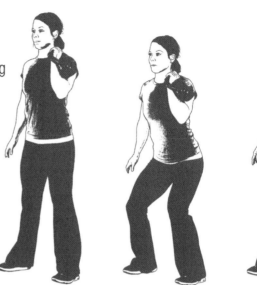

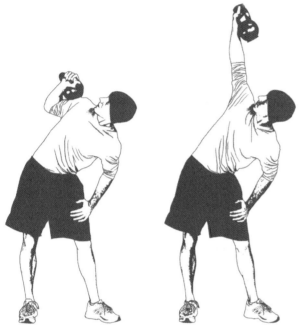

Kettlebell Side Press

- Hold a kettlebell at one shoulder and bend over toward the opposite leg.
- Use your free hand to support yourself on your thigh.
- Press the kettlebell to the ceiling, directly overhead.
- *Variation:* Try this semi-reclined on the floor or on a weight bench.

Alternating Sots Press

- Hold two kettlebells at your shoulders, while you sit in a deep squat.
- Press one kettlebell to the ceiling, letting your body rotate in the same direction.
- Lower the weight and repeat on the other side.

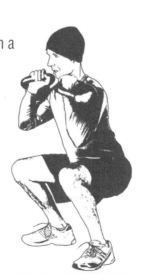
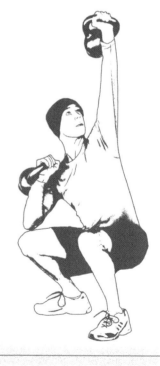

Kettlebell Upright Row

- Use two hands to grasp the handle of a kettlebell in front of your pelvis.
- Lift the kettlebell upward to your chin.
- Don't lift your elbows too high.

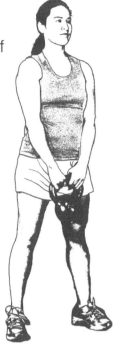
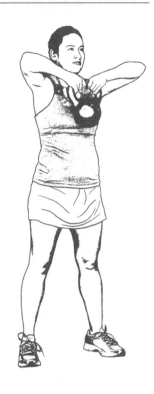

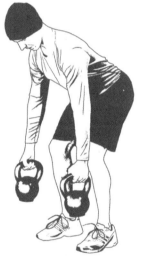
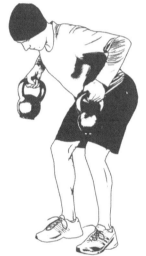

Kettlebell Double Row

- Hold two kettlebells and bend forward at your waist, while keeping your back straight.
- Pull the kettlebells up toward your chest.
- Focus on squeezing your shoulder blades together.

Kettlebell Single Bent Over Row

- Perform the same basic motion as the Kettlebell Double Row, but use a single weight.
- Place the leg on the side of the kettlebell backward a step for greater stability.
- Use your free arm to support yourself on your thigh.
- Don't let your elbow flare outward.

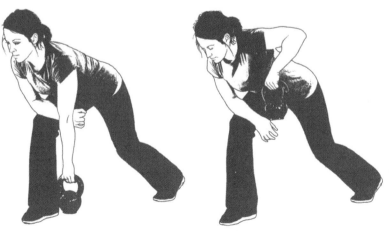

Kettlebell Iron Cross

- Raise two kettlebells overhead.
- Slowly lower the weights out to the side.
- Stop when your hands get to the height of your shoulders.
- Lift them back overhead, keeping your arms straight and out the side.
- Keep your shoulder blades pulled back and down.

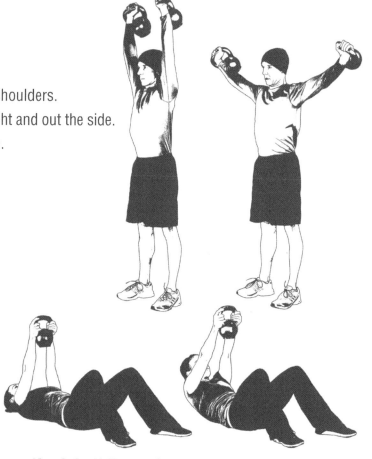

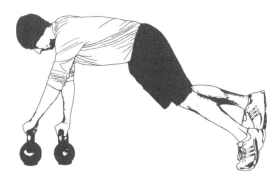

Kettlebell Bear Crawl

- Get in a quadruped position on the floor.
- Grasp two kettlebells positioned under your shoulders.
- Walk your arms forward, moving the kettlebells 8 to 12 -inches at a time.
- Advance your legs, so you crawl forward like a bear.

Kettlebell Press Crunch

- Lie on the floor, with your knees bent.
- Hold a kettlebell over your chest, with your arms extended.
- Tighten your abdominal muscles and perform a crunch, lifting the weight upward.
- *Make it harder:* Lower the weight to your chest, and then perform a chest press to raise it back to ceiling on each crunch.

Kettlebell Twisting Crunch

- Lie on the floor with one leg bent and raise a kettlebell overhead on the side with the bent leg.
- Tighten your abdominal muscles and lift your upper back from the floor.
- Press the kettlebell to the ceiling as high as you can, allowing your trunk to twist.
- Use your other hand as a counterbalance.

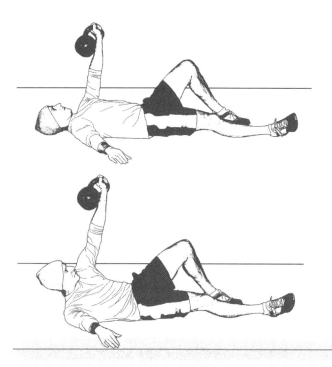

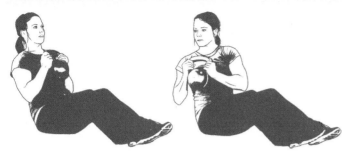

Kettlebell Russian Twist

- Sit on the floor with a slight bend in your knees.
- Hold a kettlebell at your chest.
- Rotate side to side, twisting your trunk by using your abdominal muscles.
- *Make it harder:* Keep your feet off the floor.

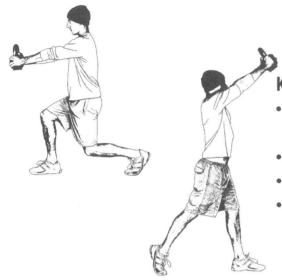

Kettlebell Reach & Twist

- Start in a split squat while holding a kettlebell over your front knee.
- Swivel on your feet to switch positions onto your opposite leg.
- Stand up and raise the kettlebell above your head.
- Rotate back to the starting position.

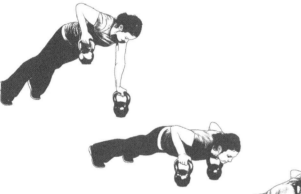

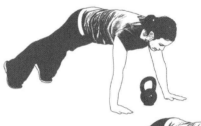

Renegade Push-up

- Assume a push-up position on the floor, holding two kettlebells under your shoulders.
- Pull one kettlebell to your chest, then lower it to the floor.
- Perform a push-up and then row the second kettlebell to your chest.

Kettlebell Ballistic Push-up

- Get in a push-up position with one hand on the body of a kettlebell.
- Drop to a push-up then explode upward and switch your hand positions.
- Jump back and forth, switching hands on each push-up.
- *Variation:* Place the kettlebell on its side so you have a more stable surface to balance on.

Chapter 6

"These are big moves and they will shape you into a more complete athlete."

Big Moves

Consider these activities: Diving to the ground to avoid being tagged in a dodge ball game. Lifting a heavy box to the upper shelf of a closet. Paddling a canoe down a stretch of white rapids.

When you imagine yourself in each of those situations, what does it feel like to move your body? Are you focused on one single motion, or are you thinking about the rapid cascade of many simultaneous actions?

Life and sport rarely happen in one plane of movement. Nor do they typically entail the use of just one body part, joint, or muscle. When we move, we use our whole bodies.

Your workouts should reflect this idea.

The 50+ skills in the coming pages are complex movements designed to challenge your whole body. To be honest, this chapter is a bit of a grab bag of exercises. The common thread is that all of the exercises involve multiple body parts and require a high degree of coordination over multiple planes of motion. Many of the illustrations reflect exercises already seen in the two previous chapters, but with dumbbells, medicine balls, and sandbags as the tools du jour.

You might feel awkward trying out some of the skills, but that is the intention. Life and sport are awkward. When you push yourself to the limits of your abilities, you get off balance. You go beyond the limits of your normal movement repertoire.

Next to switching careers to become a river guide or relocating to a farm and filling your day with hours of bailing hay and wrestling with calves, it's the type of movements in this chapter that will help you adapt to life's physical demands. These are big moves and they will shape you into a more complete athlete.

Enough said.

Go big or go home!

Plate Hold Squat

- Hold a weight plate at arms-length from your body.
- Lower into a full-depth squat while keeping your arms extended.
- Stay tight through your trunk and return to standing.

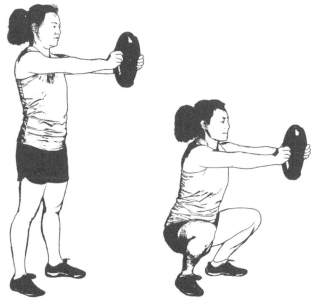

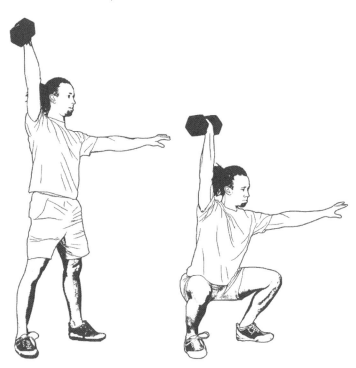

Single Arm Overhead Squat

- Use one arm to raise a single dumbbell overhead.
- Keep your arm elevated as you lower into a full-depth squat.
- Arch your back to maintain your spine curve.
- Return to standing with the dumbbell overhead.

Atlas Squat

- Balance a medicine ball on your palm with your arm raised overhead.
- Lower into a squat and let your body rotate toward the raised arm.
- Keep the ball balanced overhead and return to standing.

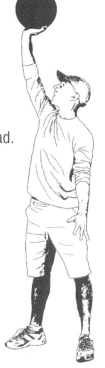

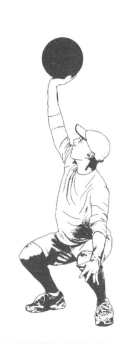

Dumbbell Overhead Squat

• Raise two dumbbells directly overhead.

• Lower into a full-depth squat.

• Arch your back to maintain your spine curve.

• Keep your arms raised as you return to standing

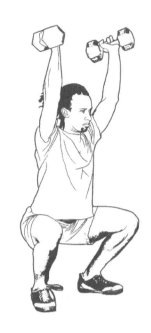

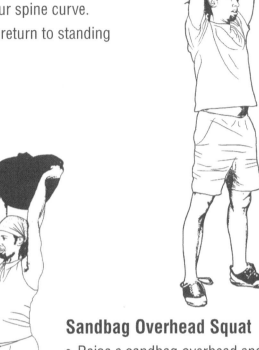

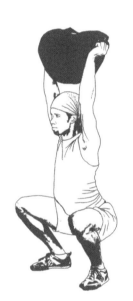

Sandbag Overhead Squat

• Raise a sandbag overhead and perform a basic Overhead Squat.

• Pull your shoulder blades together and focus on limiting excess trunk or arm motion.

Sumo Squat & Tricep Extension

• Hold two dumbbells behind your head with your elbows pointed to the ceiling.

• Lower into a Sumo Squat, with your feet nearly double shoulder-width apart and your legs rotated outward.

• As you stand-up, extend your elbows, lifting the weights to the ceiling.

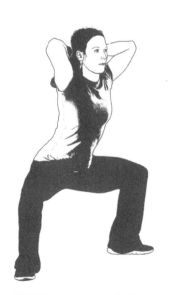

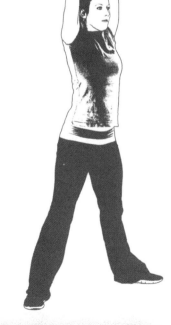

Split Squat & Shoulder Press

- Hold two dumbbells at your shoulders.
- Spread your feet apart, with one placed forward and the other behind you.
- Lower into a Split Squat.
- As you stand-up, press the dumbbells to the ceiling.

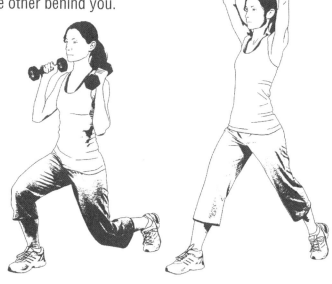

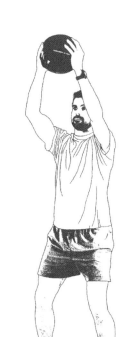

Swing Squat

- Assume a medium-depth squat, holding a medicine ball between your legs.
- Stand-up and swing the medicine ball overhead.
- Return to the squat, keeping your back arched to protect your spine.
- *Variation:* Try it with a weight plate.

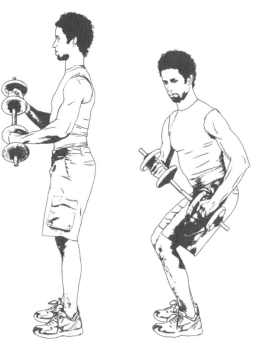

Canoe Squat

- Stand with your feet shoulder-width apart and hold two dumbbells like an oar at your side.
- Lower into a squat and "row" the dumbbells as if you were paddling a canoe.
- Return to standing between each "row" of the dumbbells.
- Alternate the side you paddle on every squat.

Wood Chop

- Use two hands to hold a medicine ball over one shoulder, near your ear.
- Drop to a squat and "chop" the weight across your body, as if you were swinging an ax.
- Keep your abdomen tight and allow your trunk to rotate in the direction of the swing.
- *Variation:* Hold a weight plate or dumbbell instead of a medicine ball.

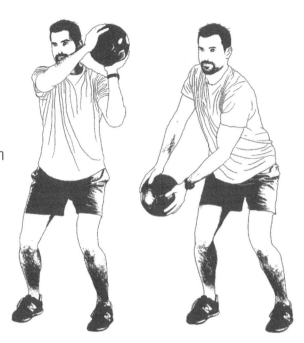

Dumbbell Thruster

- Hold two dumbbells at your shoulders with your elbows lifted.
- Drop to a squat and then explode upward.
- Thrust the dumbbells overhead as you stand-up, then lower them as you return to the squat.
- *Make it harder:* Try it with just one dumbbell or two dumbbells of different weights.

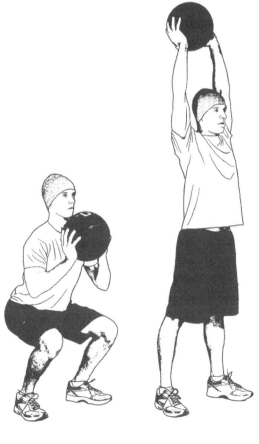

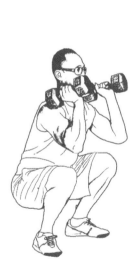

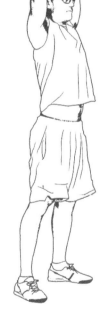

Med Ball Thruster

- Hold a medicine ball at your chest with your elbows tucked in.
- Lower to a squat and then explode upward.
- Thrust the medicine ball overhead as you stand-up, and then lower it as you return to the squat.

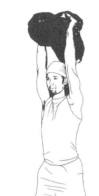
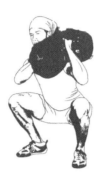

Sandbag Alternating Squat Press

- Hold a sandbag over one shoulder and lower into a squat.
- Stand up and press the sandbag directly overhead.
- Lower to a squat and bring the sandbag to rest on your opposite shoulder.
- Alternate the sandbag side to side as you squat up and down.

Wall Ball

- Face a few feet away from a wall with a medicine ball at your chest.
- Lower into a squat, keeping your elbows tucked in.
- Explode upward and throw the medicine ball as high as you can up the wall.
- Catch the medicine ball and return to a squat.

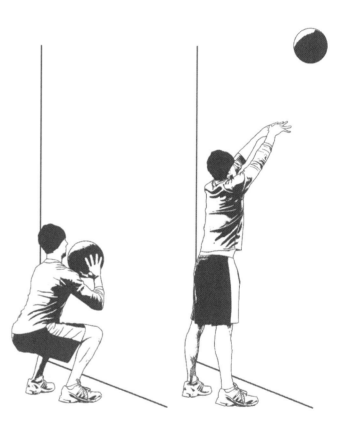

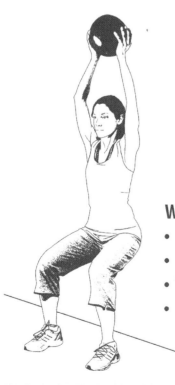

Wall Sit & Med Ball Raise

- Place your feet 18 to 24 inches away from a wall and lower into a wall sit.
- Raise a medicine ball overhead and pinch your shoulder blades together.
- Try to maintain the position for as long as you can.
- *Variation:* Use a weight plate or dumbbell instead of a medicine ball.

Scoop Throw

- Get into a squat, holding a medicine ball between your legs.
- Explode up to standing and throw the medicine ball as high as you can.
- Catch the medicine ball and return to the starting position.

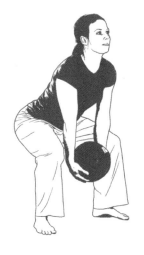
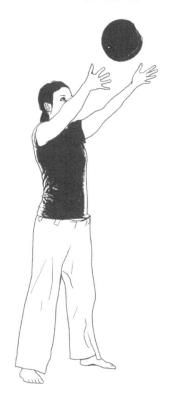

Dumbbell Swing

- Hold a single dumbbell at your thighs and lower into a partial squat.
- Stand up and swing the dumbbell forward with a straight arm.
- Lower the dumbbell as you return to the partial squat.
- *Variation:* Hold one end of the dumbbell with two hands as you swing it.

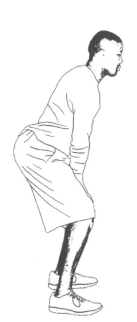
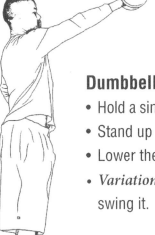
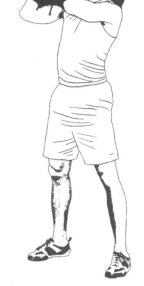

Sandbag Lift

- Straddle a sandbag placed on the floor in front of you.
- Lower into a squat and grab the sandbag with two hands.
- Stand up and swing the sandbag onto one shoulder.
- Lower it back to the ground and alternate shoulders on every lift.

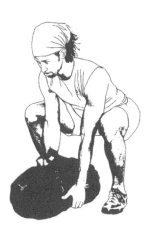

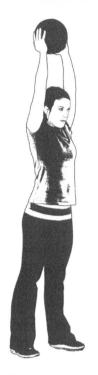

Med Ball Slam

- Raise a medicine ball overhead.
- Slam the medicine ball to the floor, throwing it down as hard as you can.
- Catch the medicine ball on its rebound and return to the starting position.

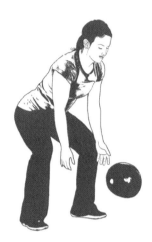

Corkscrew

- Raise a medicine ball overhead and fully twist your trunk in one direction.
- Lower the medicine ball to below your waist while dropping your body and rotating to the opposite side.
- Allow yourself to pivot on the ball of your feet for full twisting motion.
- *Variation:* Use a weight plate or dumbbell instead of a medicine ball.

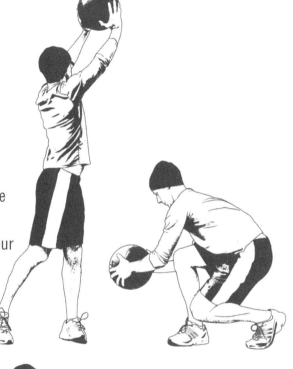

Rotating Lunge

- Hold a medicine ball at your chest.
- Take a large step forward and drop into a lunge.
- Extend your arms and rotate your trunk over the forward leg.
- Bring the medicine ball back to the middle and return to standing.

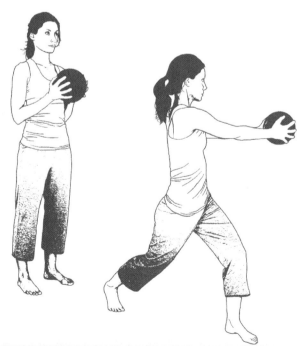

Wood Chop Lunge

- Hold a medicine ball over one shoulder, near your ear.
- Take a large step forward and drop into a lunge.
- Bring the medicine ball down toward the opposite leg in a "chopping" motion.
- Allow your trunk to rotate with the diagonal motion of your arms.
- Swing the medicine ball back to your ear and return to standing.

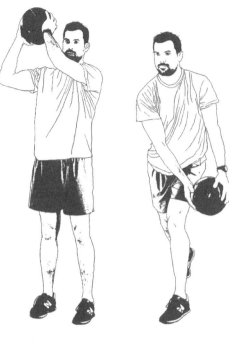

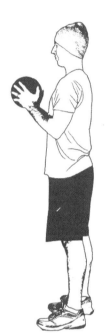

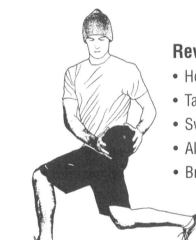

Reverse Lunge with Chop

- Hold a medicine ball at your chest.
- Take a large step backward and drop into a lunge.
- Swing the medicine ball down and over the front leg.
- Allow your trunk to rotate to the side of your front leg.
- Bring the weight back to middle and return to standing.

Reverse Lunge & Tilt

- Hold a weight plate overhead.
- Take a large step backward and drop into a lunge.
- Tilt your trunk and the weight plate over to the side of your forward leg.
- Stay tight through your abdomen and return to standing.
- *Variation:* Use a medicine ball or dumbbell.

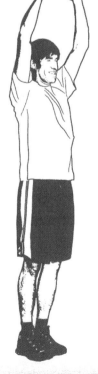

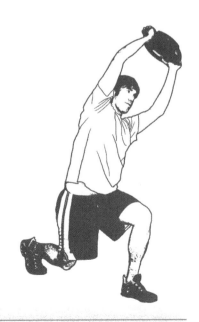

Side Lunge & Forward Raise

- Hold two dumbbells at your upper thighs.
- Take a large step out to the side and drop into a side lunge.
- Simultaneously raise both dumbbells forward to the height of your shoulders.
- Push back to the starting position and return the weights to your thighs.
- Alternate lunge to opposite side.

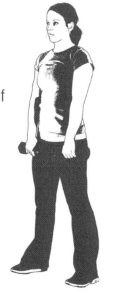
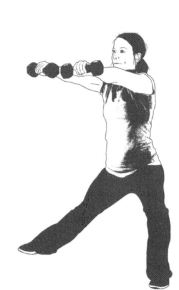

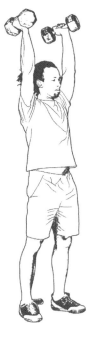
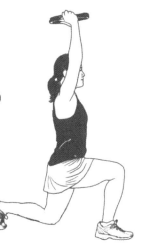

Dumbbell Overhead Lunge

- Hold two dumbbells overhead.
- Take a large step forward and drop into lunge.
- Push back to the starting position, keeping the dumbbells elevated.
- *Variation:* Hold a weight plate, medicine ball, or a single dumbbell.

Overhead Walking Lunges

- Hold a weight plate overhead and step forward into a lunge.
- Keep the weight elevated as you walk forward, lunging on each step.

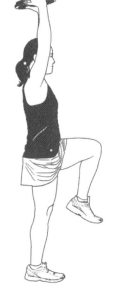
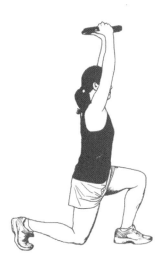

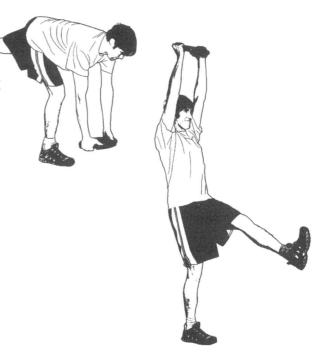

Single Leg Deadlift & Plate Raise

- Balance on a single leg, bend forward, and hold a weight plate near the floor.
- Lift your trunk and let your elevated leg swing forward.
- Raise the weight directly overhead.
- *Variation:* Try pressing the weight to the ceiling versus lifting it with straight arms.

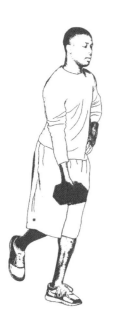
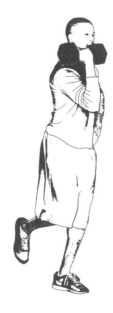

Single Leg Bicep Curl

- Balance on a single leg, holding a dumbbell over the thigh of your lifted leg.
- Curl the dumbbell to your shoulder.
- Stay tight through trunk as your curl the weight up and down.

Single Leg Row

- Balance on one leg and bend forward slightly while holding two dumbbells.
- Bring the weights to your chest in a rowing motion.
- Stay tight through your abdomen and try to minimize trunk motion.

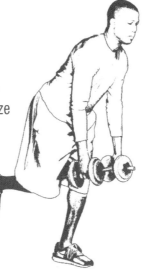
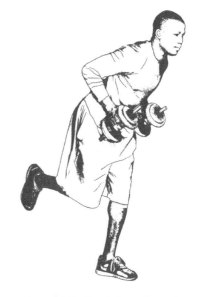

Single Leg Corkscrew

- Balance on a single leg and lower into a crouch with a medicine ball held at one side of your body.
- Stand up and bring your free leg forward while lifting the weight up and overhead.
- Allow your trunk to rotate on a diagonal as you swing the medicine ball along its path.

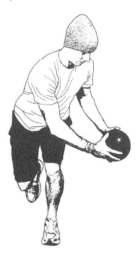
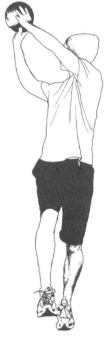

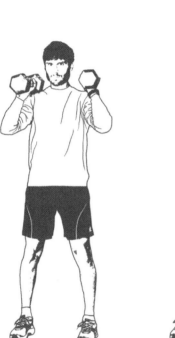
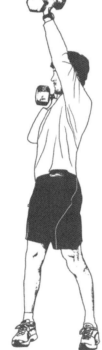

Twisting Shoulder Press

- Hold two dumbbells at your shoulders.
- Rotate to one side and press the opposite dumbbell overhead.
- Lower the weight and rotate to the other side, repeating the press with the opposite arm.

Twist & Lateral Raise

- Hold two dumbbells at your upper thighs.
- Rotate your trunk while simultaneously lifting the dumbbells outward.
- Lower the weights, rotate to the other side and lift them back up again.

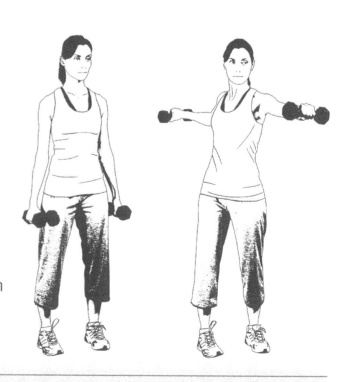

Dumbbell Toe Touch

- Stand with your feet spread nearly double shoulder-width apart.
- Hold a single dumbbell overhead.
- Bend forward and try to touch your foot with your free hand.
- Keep the dumbbell raised to the ceiling the entire time.

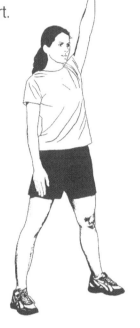
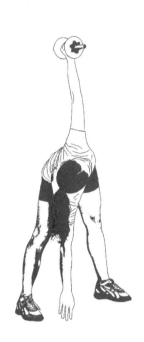

Shot Put Press

- Get in a crouched position with a dumbbell held near the shoulder of your front leg.
- Pivot on your feet to switch directions to the other side.
- Stand up and thrust the dumbbell to the ceiling, as if you were tossing a shot put.

Dumbbell Push Press

- Hold two dumbbells at your shoulders.
- Drop to a quarter-squat.
- Explode upward and press the dumbbells to the ceiling.
- *Variation:* Use a single dumbbell instead of two.

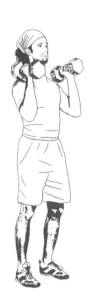
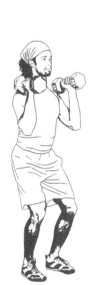
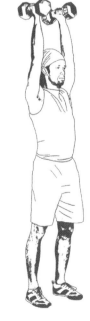

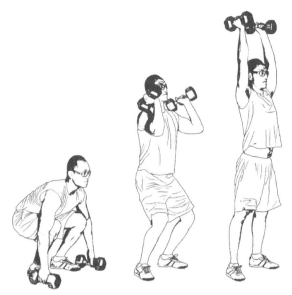

Dumbbell Clean & Press

- Reach forward to grab two dumbbells from the floor.
- Watch your knee alignment and maintain your spine curve.
- Stand up and pull both dumbbells to your shoulders.
- Immediately press the weights to the ceiling.

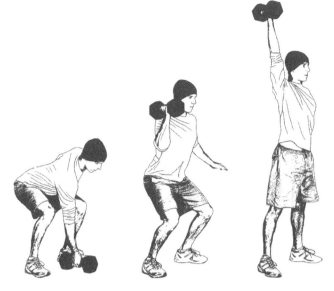

Single Arm Clean & Press

- Reach forward to grab a dumbbell from the floor.
- Keep your back arched to maintain your spine curve.
- Stand up and pull the weight to your shoulder in one motion.
- Immediately press the dumbbell to the ceiling.

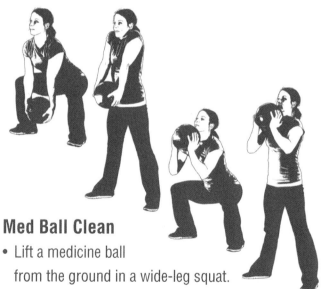

Med Ball Clean

- Lift a medicine ball from the ground in a wide-leg squat.
- Stand up and quickly pull the weight upward, shrugging your shoulders.
- Immediately drop back to a squat to catch the medicine ball at your chest.
- Return to standing, keeping the weight at your chest.

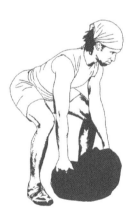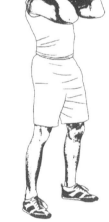

Sandbag Clean

- Bend forward to lift a sandbag from the floor.
- Arch your back to maintain your spine curve.
- Quickly stand up while pulling the sandbag up to your shoulders.
- Finish with your hips extended and your elbows lifted.
- *Variation:* Add a squat at the midpoint of the lift, as performed in the Medicine Ball Clean.

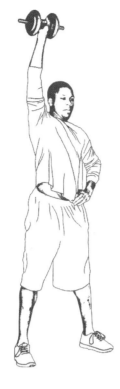
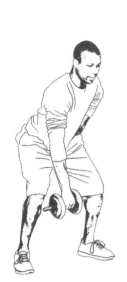

Dumbbell Hang Snatch

- Bend forward to hold a dumbbell near your shins.
- Stand up and pull the dumbbell overhead in one smooth motion.
- If necessary, add a squat at the midpoint of the lift to get under the dumbbell.
- *Variation:* Lift the dumbbell from the ground, instead of pausing at your shins.

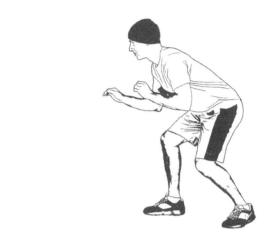

Sprawl

- Imitate the stance of a wrestler about to fight an opponent.
- Drop to the floor with your arms and legs spread, and with your belly on the ground.
- Push off the floor to jump back to the starting position.

Burpee

- Drop to the ground in a push-up position.
- Hop your feet forward, landing in a low squat.
- Explode upward, jumping into the air with your hands raised.
- *Variation:* Hold a medicine ball throughout the movement.

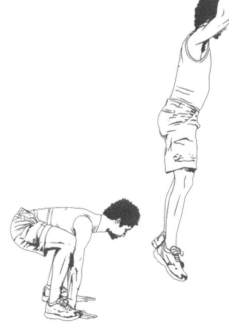
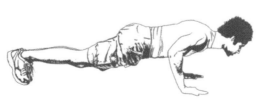

Dumbbell Burpee

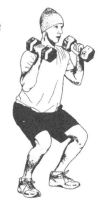
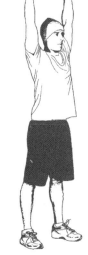

- Place two dumbbells on the ground and get in a push-up position.
- Hop to a partial squat and bring the dumbbells to your shoulders.
- Stand up and immediately thrust the dumbbells to the ceiling.
- *Make it harder:* Row each dumbbell to your shoulders when you are in the push-up position prior to jumping upward.

Sandbag Get-up

- Lie on the floor with a sandbag held near one shoulder.
- Bend the leg of the side with the sandbag while pushing yourself to sit.
- Bring your extended leg backward to get in a kneeling position.
- Keep the sandbag at your shoulder as you rise to standing.

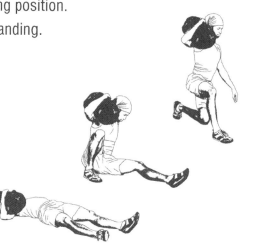

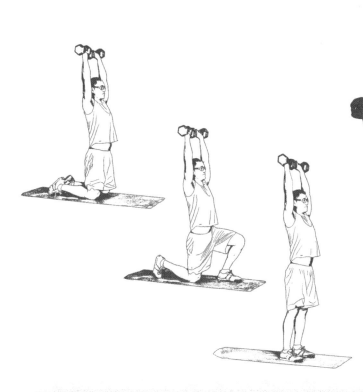

Kneeling Overhead Dumbbell Get-up

- Kneel on the floor with two dumbbells held overhead.
- Step one leg forward and push the ground to rise to standing.
- Keep the dumbbells elevated the entire time.

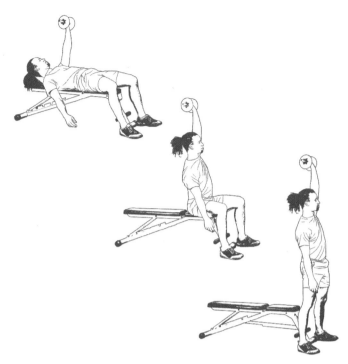

Overhead Bench Get-up

- Lie on a weight bench with a dumbbell held toward the ceiling.
- Lift your trunk to a sitting position.
- Keep moving forward to rise into standing while holding the weight overhead.
- *Make it harder:* Hold two dumbbells overhead.

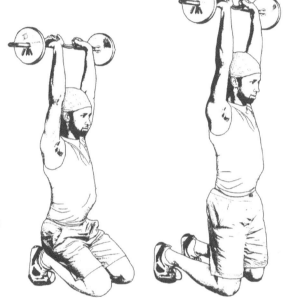

Kneeling Overhead Thrust

- Kneel on the floor and hold a barbell or two dumbbells overhead with extended arms.
- Tighten your thighs and bottom to lift your torso upward, off your heels.
- Lower back down while keeping the weight overhead.

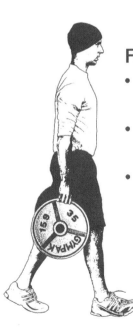

Farmer Walk

- Hold two weight plates or dumbbells at your sides.
- Walk forward and keep your chest elevated.
- Stay tight through your abdomen and relax your shoulders.

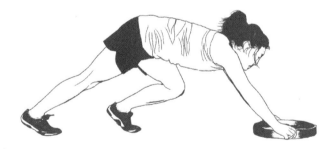

Plate Push

- Place both hands on a weight plate resting on the ground.
- Extend your legs behind you.
- Drive the weight plate forward by pushing through your feet.

Chapter 7

"It's so simple – but that's the beauty of the push-up."

Mad Push-ups

Start in a plank position, balanced on your toes with your arms extended beneath your shoulders. Drop your sternum to the floor before firing your chest and triceps to push back to the plank. Stay tight across your trunk throughout the motion.

It's so simple—but that's the beauty of the push-up.

Everyone from gym teachers to boxing trainers go gaga for push-ups. You can do them in the garage, next to your bed, on the beach, and even at work if you feel the urge. No equipment is required and they challenge everything from your arms, chest, core, and hips.

Does the push-up deserve the title of the most fundamental body-weight exercise in the world? Perhaps. Does the push-up deserve its own chapter? Absolutely.

If you mix up your hand and feet position, plus throw in a few simple props, you can come up with dozens of different push-up variations. Luckily for you, I've spared you the time it takes to brainstorm the different varieties: This chapter has over 40 different push-up positions and movements.

I doubt you're the type of person that ever gets bored in your workouts, but with this plethora of push-up variations, you'll never be able to use that excuse again!

Push-up

- Begin with your hands on the ground, arms straight, legs extended, and body balanced on your tiptoes.
- Bend your elbows and lower your sternum to the floor.
- Stay tight through your trunk and don't let your elbows flare out to the side.
- Push the floor and straighten your arms to return to the starting position.

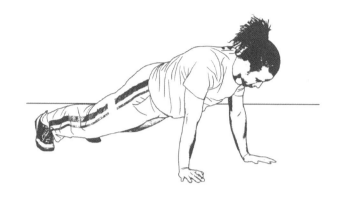

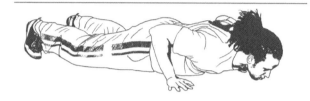

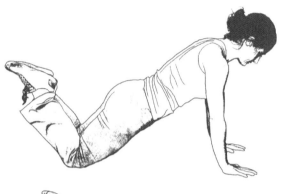

Knee Push-up

- Place your knees on the floor and balance with your arms extended beneath your trunk.
- Bend your elbows to lower your chest to the floor.
- Don't let your abdomen sag downward.
- Push the floor and straighten your arms to return to the starting position.

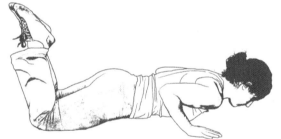

Wall Push-up

- Stand with your feet 24 to 36 inches (or more) away from a wall.
- Place your palms on the wall at chest height.
- Bend your elbows to lower your chest to the wall.
- Press the wall and extend your arms to return to the starting position.

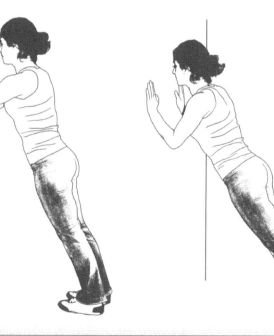

Chair Push-up

- Place your hands on a sturdy chair and extend your legs behind you.
- Lower your chest to the chair.
- Push through your arms to return to the starting position.
- Stay tight through your core and lower body.

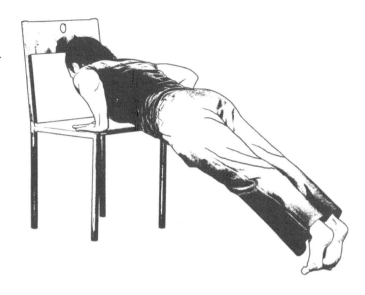

Countertop Push-up

- Place your hands on the edge of a countertop and extend your legs a few feet behind you.
- Lower your sternum to the counter without letting your abdomen sag.
- Push the counter and straighten your arms to return to the starting position.

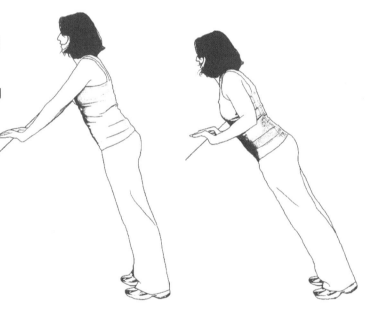

Wide Push-up

- Spread your hands double shoulder-width on the floor and get into the basic Push-up position.
- Lower your body to the floor, then press back up to the starting position.

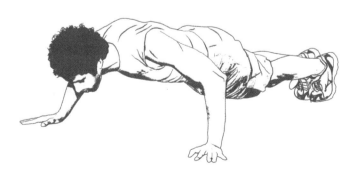

Narrow Grip Push-up

- Place your hands nearly together and centered beneath your chest.
- Lower yourself to the floor, then press back up to the starting position.
- Keep your elbows tucked into your ribs as much as possible.

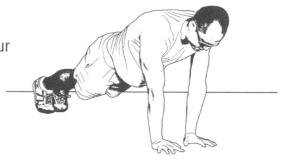

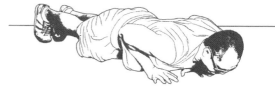

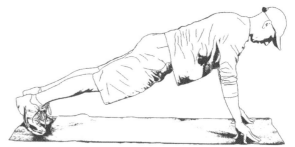

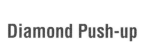

Diamond Push-up

- Place your thumbs and index fingers together on the floor, forming a diamond with your hands.
- Lower your chest to the floor, staying tight through your trunk.
- Press back up to the starting position.

Fist Push-up

- Place your two fists on the ground, resting on your knuckles.
- Stay tight across your wrists so they don't buckle underneath you.
- Lower down and back up through a push-up, without bending your wrists.

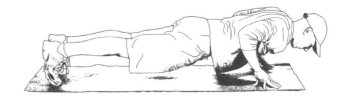

Fingertip Push-up

- Balance on your fingertips in the starting position of a basic Push-up.
- Lower yourself down and back up while staying elevated on your fingertips.

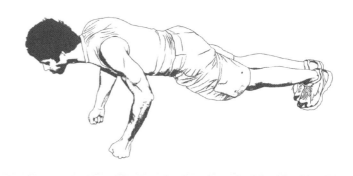

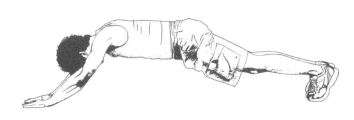

Overhead Push-up

- Place your hands on the floor at or above the position of your head.
- Stay tight across your trunk in this elongated plank position.
- Lower your trunk to the floor by bending your elbows, then press back up to the starting position.
- *Variation:* Play with having your hands spread wide versus almost touching.

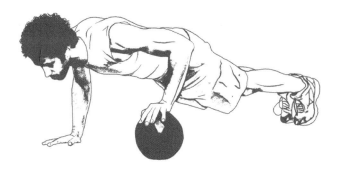

Uneven Push-up

- Place one hand on a medicine ball or another elevated surface with your other hand directly on the floor.
- Perform a basic Push-up motion with your hands in this uneven placement.
- Don't let either elbow flare too far out to the side.

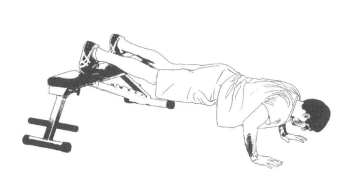

Decline Push-up

- Place your feet on a weight bench, stair, or another elevated surface.
- Lower your chest to the floor while you stay tight across your trunk and hips.
- Press back up to the starting position.
- *Make it harder:* Lift one foot off the bench.

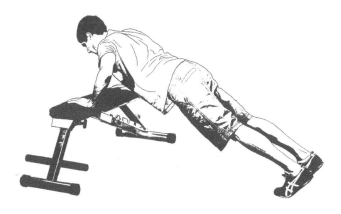

Incline Push-up

- Place your hands on a weight bench, plyo box, or another elevated surface.
- Extend your feet behind you in a basic Push-up position.
- Lower your chest to the bench, then press back up to the starting position.

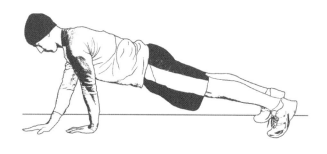

Inline Push-up

- Place your hands beneath your chest along a line on the floor, with the fingers of one hand pointing to the palm of your other hand.
- Maintain this hand placement and complete a basic Push-up movement.

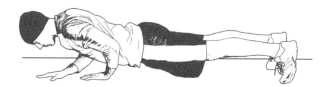

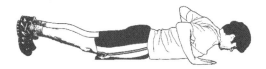

Push-up "Plus"

- Assume a basic Push-up position on the floor with normal hand and foot placement.
- Lower your chest to the floor, then press back up.
- Instead of stopping at the starting position, keep pressing your chest upward to spread your shoulder blades apart.

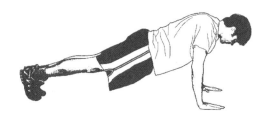

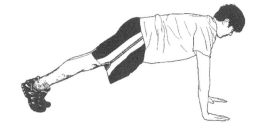

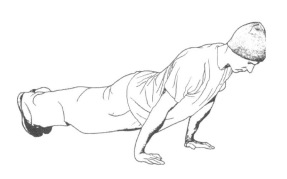

Pseudo Planche Push-Up

- Place your hands beneath your torso, positioned very low, near the bottom of your ribs.
- Shift your shoulders forward as far as you can and lower your chest to the floor.
- Return to the starting position while keeping your weight shifted as far forward as you can.
- *Make it harder:* Place your feet on a bench to shift greater weight into your shoulders.

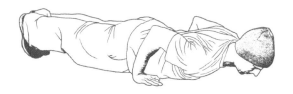

Outrigger Push-up

- Get on the floor with one hand underneath your chest and the other hand positioned off to the side, elevated on a ball or stack of weights.
- Extend your legs behind you and maintain your hand positions as you move down and up through a push-up motion.
- *Variation:* Try to balance your outer hand on just your fingertips.

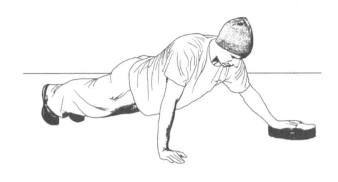

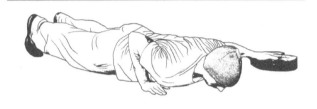

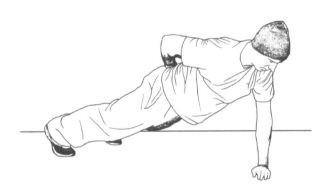

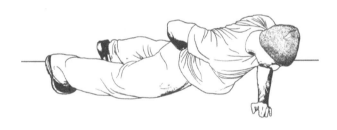

One Arm Push-up

- Place one hand on the floor underneath your chest with your fingers pointed inward.
- Keep your other hand off the floor, preferably tucked behind your back.
- Stay tight through your trunk and lower your body to the floor.
- Push hard through your bottom hand to press back up to the starting position.

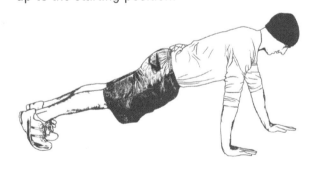

Staggered Push-up

- Spread your hands apart on the ground with one placed above your shoulders and the other beneath your shoulders.
- Maintain this hand position and lower your chest to the floor.
- Press back up to the starting position.

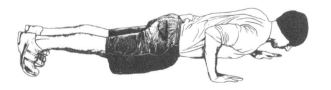

Med Ball Push-up

- Place both hands on a medicine ball, directly under your sternum.
- Balance on the ball and lower your chest downward.
- Touch your chest to the ball, then press back up to the starting position.

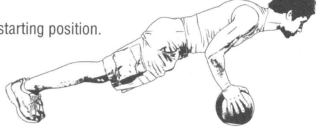

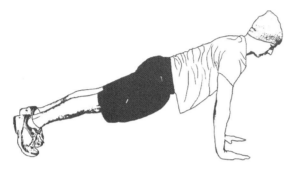

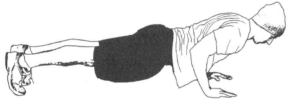

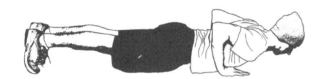

Triple Stop Push-up

- Assume a basic Push-up position on the floor
- Lower your body halfway to the floor and pause.
- Lower your chest the rest of the way and pause a second time.
- Press back halfway to the starting position and pause a third time.
- Finish by raising all the way back up.

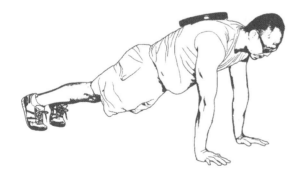

Weighted Push-up

- Get on the floor in a basic Push-up position.
- Place a weight plate on your back, centered over your shoulders.
- Perform a push-up while balancing the weight on your back.

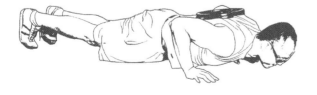

Reverse Grip Push-up

- Get on the floor in a basic Push-up position, but with your hands rotated backward.
- Lower your chest to the floor, then press back to the start.
- *Make it harder:* Elevate your feet behind you on a weight bench or stair.

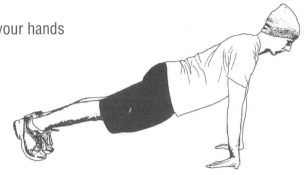

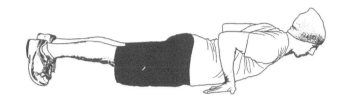

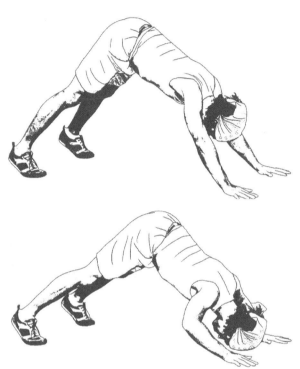

Pike Push-up

- Get on the floor with your butt in the air and your hands and feet spread shoulder-width apart.
- Keep your hips elevated and bend your elbows to lower your head to the floor.
- Straighten your arms to press back to the starting position.

Plank Press-up

- Lie on the ground with elbows bent and forearms flat against the floor.
- Press through your hands and straighten your arms to lift your body toward the ceiling.
- Lower your elbows to the floor and come to rest on your forearms again.

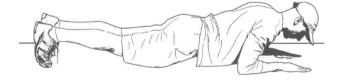

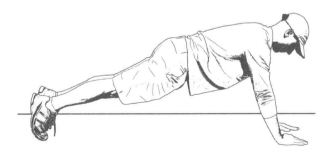

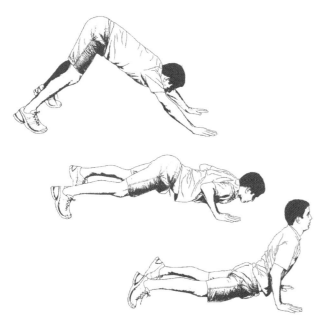

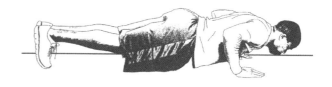

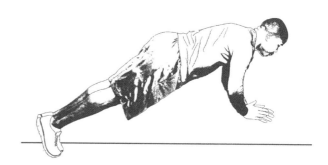

Dive Bomber Push-Up

- Get in the starting position for a Pike Push-up.
- Bend your elbows and drive your chest downward between your hands.
- Keep your momentum moving forward and push your chest upward, lifting your head to the ceiling.
- Reverse the movement, dropping back to the floor and pushing backward to the pike position.

Plyo Push-up

- Get on the floor in a basic Push-up position.
- Drop to the floor, then explode upward completely lifting your hands from the ground.
- Catch the ground softly and return to the starting position.
- *Make it harder:* Clap your hands or try to slap your thighs.

Drop Push-up

- Place your hands on two low boxes spread greater than shoulder-width apart.
- The rest of your body should be in a basic Push-up position.
- Quickly push off from the boxes and drop to the ground, gently lowering your chest to the floor.
- Explode upward so that you replace your hands on top of the boxes.

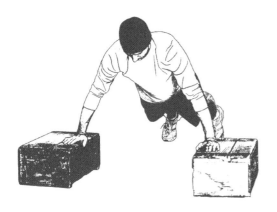

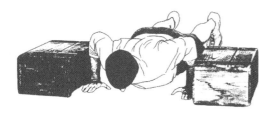

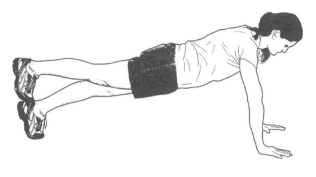

Stacked Feet Push-up

- Get in a basic Push-up position, but place the toes of one foot on the heel of the other.
- Hold this foot arrangement while you move down and up through a push-up motion.

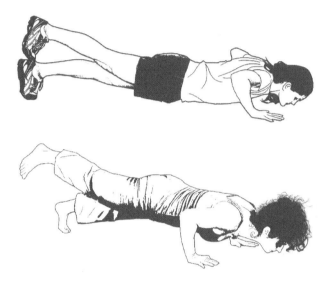

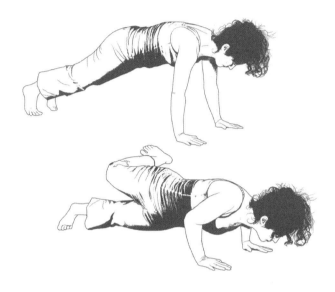

Single Leg Push-up

- Get on the ground in a Push-up position, but hold one foot 6 to 12 inches off the floor.
- Keep your leg elevated while you move down and up through a push-up motion.

Scorpion Push-up

- Assume a basic Push-up position on the floor with your feet and hands placed in normal alignment.
- As you lower your chest to the floor, lift one leg and kick it upward and over the opposite leg.
- *Make it harder*: Keep your leg lifted in the scorpion position throughout the movement.

Spiderman Push-up

- Get on the floor in a Push-up position, but keep one leg off the ground, flexed at the knee and hip.
- Lower your chest to the ground while bringing the elevated leg to your elbow.
- Allow your trunk to side bend (crunch) as your knee and elbow come together.

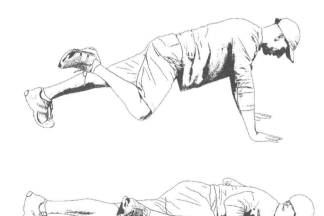

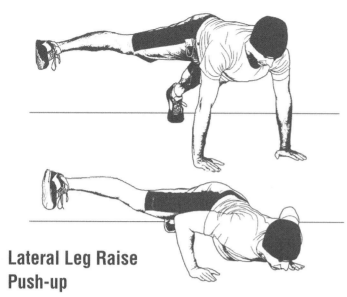

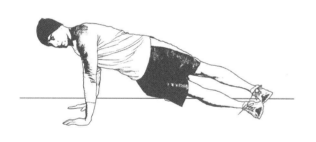

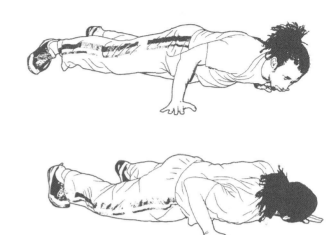

Lateral Leg Raise Push-up

- Get on the floor in a Push-up position, but lift one leg out to the side.
- Lower your chest to the floor then press back to the start.
- Keep your leg straight and hold it 6 to 12 inches off the ground through out the movement.

Side to Side Push-up

- Assume a Push-up position on the floor.
- Lower your chest to the ground.
- Before pressing back to the ceiling, shift your weight from one hand to the other, allowing your shoulder to drop toward each wrist.

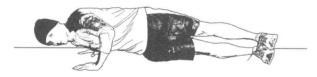

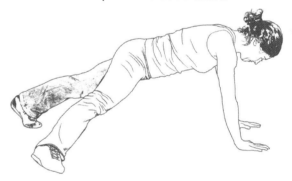

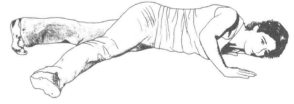

Rotated Push-up

- Stack your feet on top of each other with your heels and arches touching.
- Place your hands on the ground while keeping your lower body rotated sideways.
- Stay in this twisted position and lower your chest to the floor, then press back to the starting position.

Leg Twist Push-up

- Get on the floor in a Push-up position, but place one leg out to the side resting on the inner foot.
- Lower your chest to the floor while letting your trunk rotate to the side of the outward placed leg.
- Press back to the starting position.

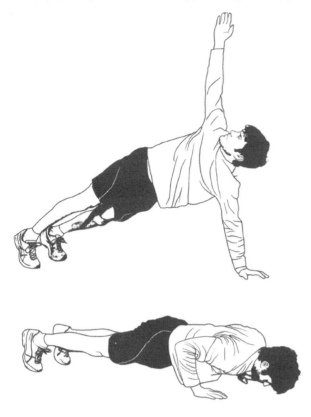

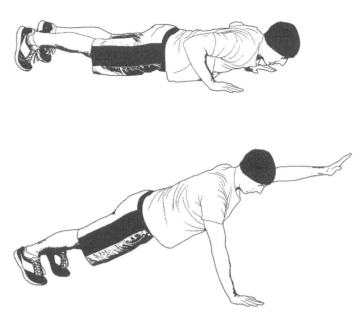

"T" Push-up

- Start in a basic Push-up position and lower your chest to the floor.
- As you return upward, lift one hand to the side and rotate your trunk until your arm is completely above you.
- Bring the hand back to the ground and alternate sides with each push-up.

Push-up Arm Raise

- Lower your chest to the floor with a basic Push-up technique.
- As you press yourself upward, swing one hand toward the ceiling.
- Place the hand back on the ground and alternate arms on each repetition.
- *Make it harder:* Throw both hands to the ceiling, then catch the ground softly and return to the starting position.

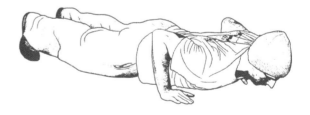

Backward Push-up

- Get on the floor in a basic Push-up position.
- Lower your chest to the floor.
- Press yourself backward into a supported crouch as you raise your chest off the floor.
- Return to the starting position.

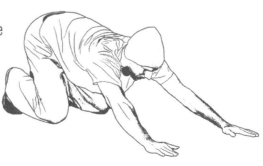

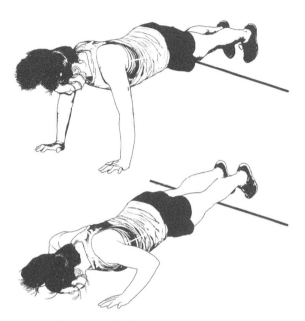

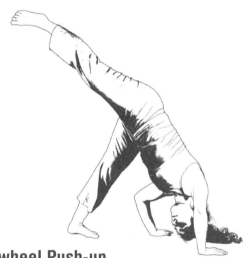

Elevated Feet Wall Push-up

• Place both feet against a wall, 12 inches above the floor.
• Lower your body down into a push-up while keeping your legs pressed against the wall.
• Stay tight in your trunk and don't let your abdomen sag downward.

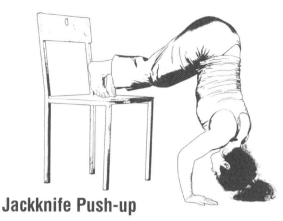

Jackknife Push-up

• Place your feet on a chair or box.
• Hinge forward 90 degrees from your trunk to place your hands on the ground directly beneath your shoulders.
• Bend your elbows to lower your head to the floor, then press back to the starting position.

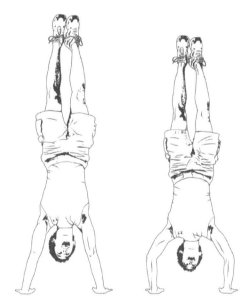

Cartwheel Push-up

• Bend forward from your waist to place both hands on the ground, beneath your shoulders.
• Raise one leg up in the air as if you were going to kick-over into a cartwheel.
• Bend your arms to lower your head to the floor, then press back up to the starting position.

Handstand Push-up

• Kick up to a handstand against a wall, with your hands beneath your shoulders.
• Bend your elbows to lower your head to the floor, and then return to the starting position.
• Stay tight through your trunk so you don't arch your back too much.
• *Variation:* Face the wall instead of having your back against it.

Breakdance Push-up

- Crouch in a low squat with your hands in front of your body.
- Reach forward to place both palms on the ground, angled off-center from your trunk.
- Lower your head and one shoulder to the floor while lifting your legs off the ground and balancing on your hands.
- Explode backward to get your feet on the ground and return to the starting position.

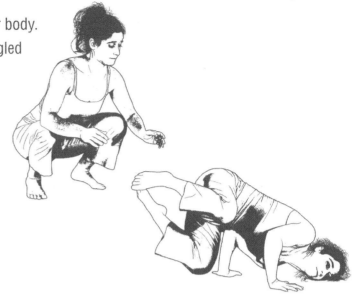

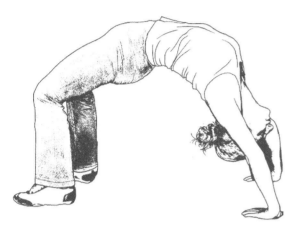

Backbend Push-up

- Get on the ground in a backbend with your spine arched and your hips raised to the ceiling.
- Bend your elbows to carefully lower your head to the ground.
- Maintain the backbend and straighten your arms to return to the starting position.
- *Make it harder*: Lift one leg off the ground, holding it to the ceiling.

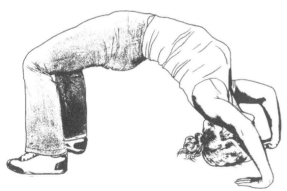

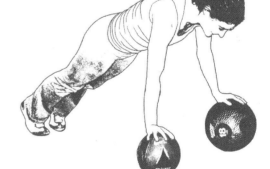

Double Med Ball Push-up

- Place your hands on two medicine balls beneath your shoulders with your legs extended beneath you.
- Maintain your balance as you lower your chest downward.
- Press back up to the starting position.

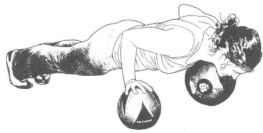

Chapter 8

"There is a simple and addictive joy in being able to lift yourself through space in awkward positions."

Monkey Style

Weight lifting with dumbbells, barbells, and other iron is a time-tested way to build strength, but it's a stretch of the imagination to call it fun. And bragging about how much weight you can lift is a quick way to bore your friends. Contrast that with gymnastics-type strength: Learning new gymnastics skills is both entertaining and cause for serious pride. There is a simple and addictive joy in being able to lift yourself through space in awkward positions. More importantly, mastering body-weight gymnastics skills is a fundamental pathway to becoming a better athlete.

Raising your body to an overhead surface. Holding a static position for an extended time. Exploding off the floor. Suspending your weight from an overhang. These movements don't just apply to circus performers or obstacle course racers. The greater control you can command over your body, the better prepared you are to respond to any physical challenge. Gymnastics conditioning is the perfect supplement your pursuit of fitness and athletic prowess.

Instead of a movement progression culminating in handsprings, flips, and other inversions, this chapter focuses on the type of basic exercises that gymnasts and other acrobats use to achieve their monkey-like strength. You'll find moves that are performed on rings, pull-up bars, and mini parallel bars, called parallettes. There are also a handful of skills performed directly on the ground, with a plyo box, or a railing. However, you really don't need any fancy equipment. If you don't have rings or space in your home for a pull-up bar, the play structure at your neighborhood park will allow you to do over 90% of the moves.

As with all body-weight strength training, for gymnastics-type conditioning you need to pay attention to other measures than how much weight you are lifting. First and foremost, you must try to execute perfect form with each skill. After you have mastery of the basic motion, then you can start to go for multiple repetitions of a movement or to hold the position for longer and longer durations. Once you can crank out a crazy number of repetitions or you get bored with how long you can hold a position, it's time to up the ante and move on to a harder movement.

You might be surprised that some of the movements have little resemblance to classic strength training and really look like basic acrobatics. Good eye. Movements like the shoulder roll, kip-up, rail walk, and vault aren't designed to make you stronger per se, but they have an important place in helping you become a well-rounded athlete. Rather than making you faster, they will challenge your coordination, ultimately molding you into a better human animal.

Finally, it goes without saying that caution should be used for any skill that is performed upside-down. Be safe and have a buddy act as a spotter the first time you work on a new movement. Train smart today so you can live to play another day!

Handstand Kick-up

- Place your hands on the floor along a wall.
- Kick your legs overhead to achieve a handstand against the wall.
- Lower one leg at a time back to the floor slowly.
- *Make it harder:* Don't use a wall.

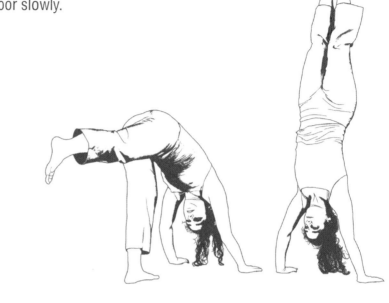

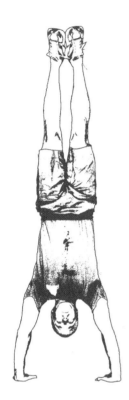

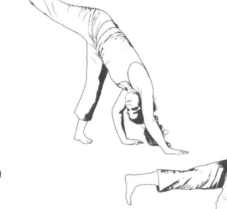

Handstand

- Kick up to a handstand and hold the position for time.
- Tighten your abdomen and buttocks to maintain your trunk straight.

Handstand Kick-over

- Place your hands on the floor.
- Shift your weight onto your arms and raise one leg from the floor as if you were doing a cartwheel.
- Kick your opposite leg upward so both feet are spread apart in the air.
- Drop your first leg to the floor and shift your weight onto that leg.
- Hop back and forth from one side to the other.

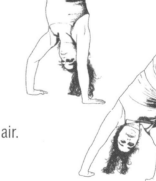

Handstand Walk

- Assume a Handstand position on the floor.
- Tighten your abdomen and buttocks to maintain your trunk straight.
- Keep your feet in the air and walk your hands forward as far as you can go.

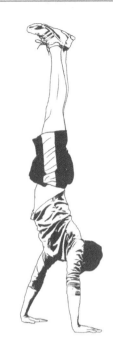

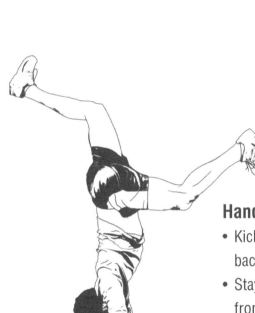

Handstand Scissors

- Kick up to a Handstand, but let your legs spread apart front to back.
- Stay balanced on your hands while you scissor-kick your legs front to back.
- Try to keep this position and your legs moving for as long as you can.

Headstand Leg Raise

- Place your head and hands on the ground in a tripod position.
- Raise your legs overhead into a headstand position.
- Stay tight through your trunk.
- Slowly lower your feet to the floor, and then raise them back to vertical.

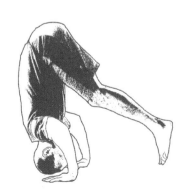

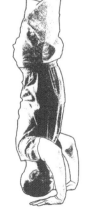

Press Handstand

- Place your hands on the ground (away from a wall) with your feet spread apart in the semi-splits.
- Shift your weight forward onto your hands and begin to pull your feet inward and toward your hands.
- Start lifting your feet from the ground and keep them moving upward until you achieve a full handstand.

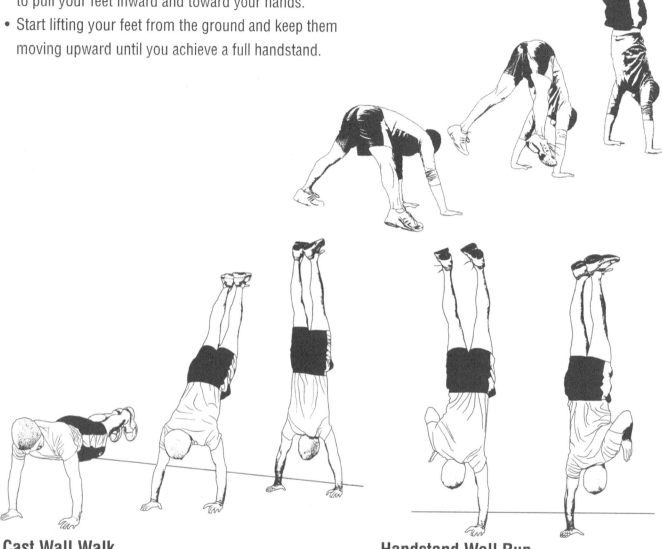

Cast Wall Walk

- Get in a Push-up position with your feet against a wall.
- Walk your hands inward to the wall and let your feet inch upward.
- Keep moving your chest toward the wall until you are in a full handstand.
- Walk your hands outward and let your feet slide down to the starting position.

Handstand Wall Run

- Get in a handstand with your chest toward a wall.
- Shift your weight to one arm and lift the other to bring your hand upward to your shoulder.
- March with your hands from side to side, bringing each hand up to the shoulder.
- *Make it harder:* Try to slap your thigh with your free arm.

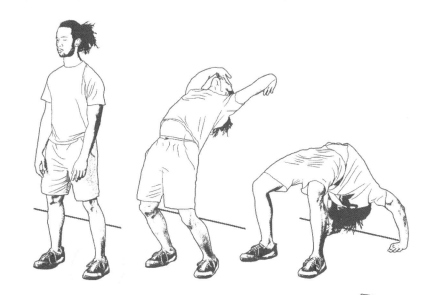

Backward Wall Walk

- Stand about 2 to 3 feet away from a wall, facing away from it.
- Reach your arms overhead and arch backward to touch the wall.
- Stay tight in your abdomen and walk your hands down the wall to the floor.
- Walk your hands back up and return to the starting position.

Deck Squat

- Lie on your back and raising your knees and arms into the air.
- Throw your arms and legs downward, using momentum to bring you forward into a low squat.
- Straighten your legs to rise to a full standing position.

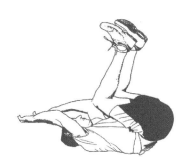
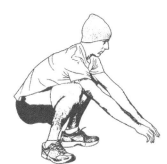
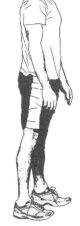

Kip-up

- Lie on your back and place your hands by your head.
- Lift your knees and hips toward your chest.
- Kick your legs up and forward as hard as you can, propelling yourself off the ground.
- Land on your feet and straighten to a standing position.

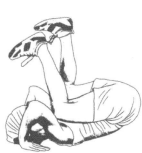
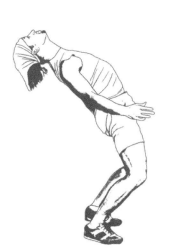
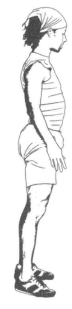

Bridge-up

- Lie on your back with your knees bent and hands placed near your ears.
- Tighten your trunk and push into your feet and hands, driving your belly toward the ceiling.
- Straighten your arms and legs as much as you can, before returning to the floor.

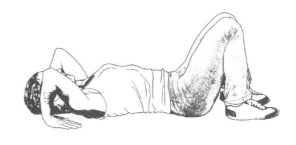

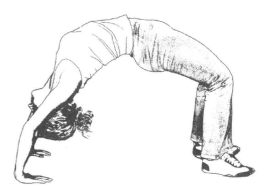

Shoulder Roll

- Place your hands and forearms on the floor in the shape of a triangle.
- Lower one shoulder to the floor and shift your weight forward.
- Keep your weight going forward and roll across your back in a diagonal line.
- Step out of the roll one leg at a time and come up to stand.

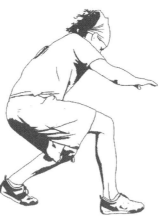

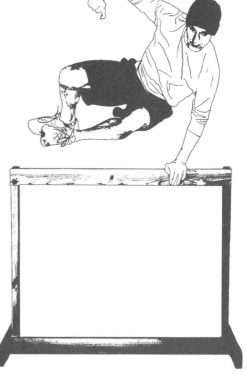

Vault

- Use a low wall, fence, or stack of mats as an obstacle.
- Place one hand on top and hop your body over.
- Jump back and forth without touching your feet to the obstacle.

Cocorinha Squat

- Squat down to a tripod position with an outstretched arm placed on the ground behind you.
- Hold this low squat and raise your opposite arm overhead.
- Shift your weight forward and return to standing.
- Alternate which hand you place on the ground.
- *This is a defensive movement from capoeira and a great exercise for flexibility and leg strength.*

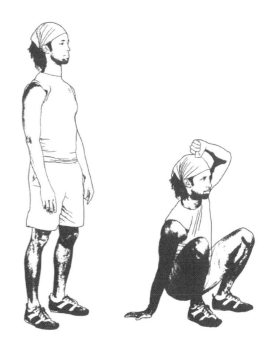

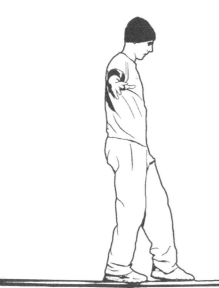

Rail Walk

- Challenge your balance by walking across a low rail or narrow balance beam.
- Try to stay on the rail for as long as you can.
- *Make it harder:* Add 180-degree turns or try side-stepping.

Rail Squat

- Balance sideways on a low rail or narrow balance beam.
- Keep your weight in the balls of your feet and lower down into a squat.
- Let your arms rise forward as a counterbalance.
- Return to standing without losing your balance.

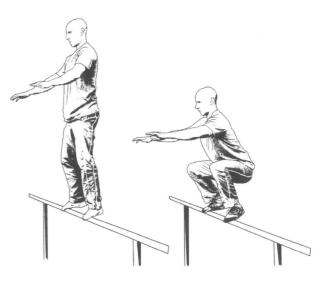

Cat Walk

- Balance in a quadruped position on a low railing.
- Advance your hands and feet while staying low and keeping your back flat.
- *Variation:* Hold one position for as long as you can and lift one arm or leg.

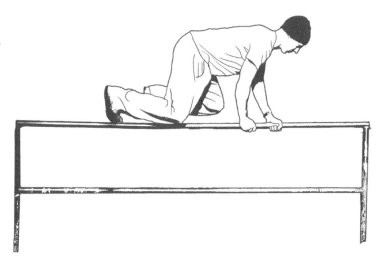

Precision Jumps

- Use two lines or boards as targets on the ground.
- Perform a standing broad jump from one to the other.
- Land softly on the balls of your feet and try to maintain your balance.

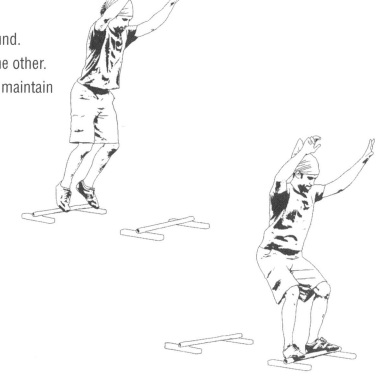

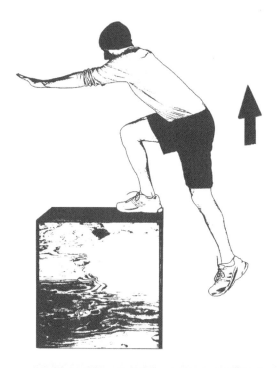

Big Step-up

- Find a large plyo box or small set of stairs.
- Place one foot on the top of the box or stairs.
- Shift your weight forward and straighten your leg to stand up.
- Lower back down to the floor.

Box Jump

- Stand 12 to 24 inches away from a plyo box.
- Bend your knees slightly, and then jump to the top of the box.
- Land softly and straighten your legs to stand up.
- Hop back to the floor as quietly as possible.

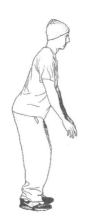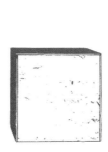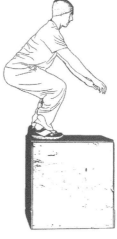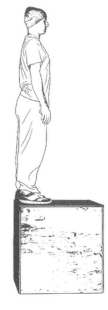

Depth Jump

- Stand on the top of a bench or a plyo box.
- Jump to the ground and immediately spring upward again.
- Try to jump as far forward as you can, but land as softly as possible.

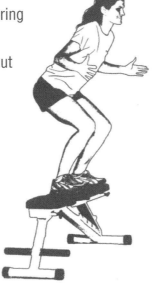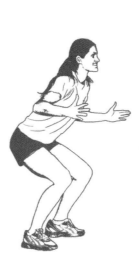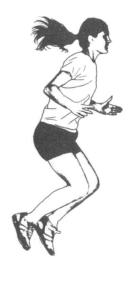

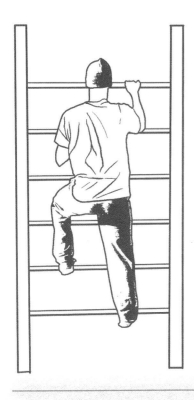

Climb

- Climb anything you can find: a tree, ladder, rope.
- Be sure that you can climb back down safely.
- *Make it harder:* Wear a weight vest or go for speed.

Brachiate

- Find an elevated beam or a set of overhead bars to hang from.
- Swing your body and walk your arms forward one at a time.
- Try not to match your hand placements (reach as far forward as you can).

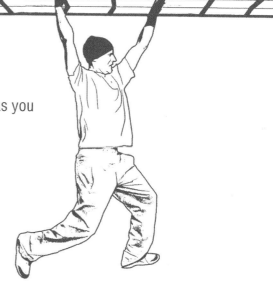

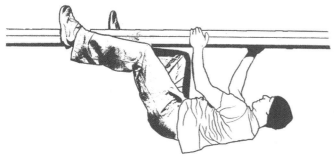

Ninja Crawl

- Hang on the underside of a beam or rail, using your arms and legs for support.
- Advance your hands and feet so you move forward along the beam.
- Try to go as far as you can.

Dip

- Place your hands on a set of parallel bars or the back of two chairs for support.
- Suspend your trunk above the bars by fully extending your arms and letting your legs dangle beneath you.
- Allow your elbows to bend and lower your chest toward your hands.
- Maintain a neutral position in your neck.
- Press through your arms to return to the starting position.

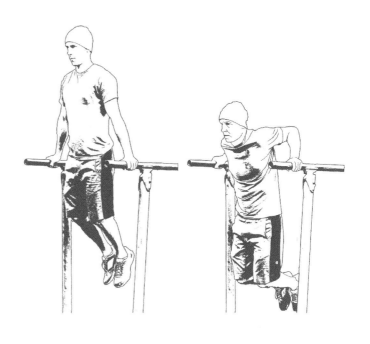

Wall Dip

- Position your upper body over the top of a wall, with your hands placed at your sides and your legs dangling beneath you.
- Lower your sternum to the wall, keeping your elbows tucked into your ribs.
- Push through your elbows to raise your chest back to the starting position.

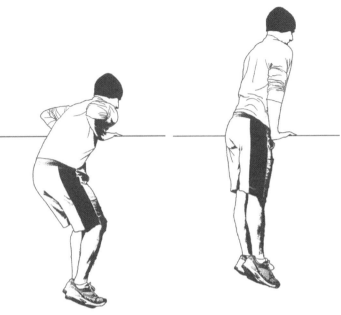

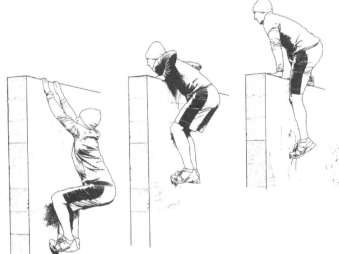

Wall Climb

- Hang from an overhead wall, supported by your hands and feet.
- Pull yourself to the top of the wall, shifting your chest over your hands.
- Press your arms into full extension, lifting your chest off the wall.
- Finish by getting your feet on the wall and standing all the way up.

Human Flag

- Grab a vertical bar, like a stop sign or lamppost, using two hands in a wide grip.
- Tighten your shoulders and trunk, and then lift your legs off the ground.
- Raise your legs higher than your trunk, then let them lower to horizontal.
- Hold the position for as long as you can.

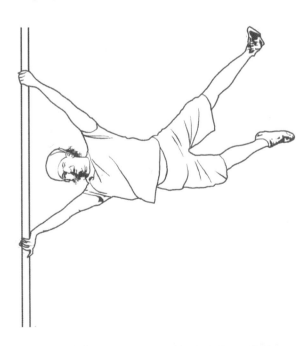

Dragon Flag

- Lie on the ground and hold onto a low railing positioned above your head.
- Tighten your shoulders and trunk, and then raise your lower body off the floor.
- Stay straight through your body and try to hold your legs off the floor in this position for as long as you can.

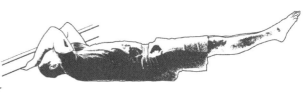

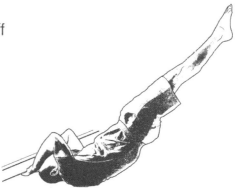

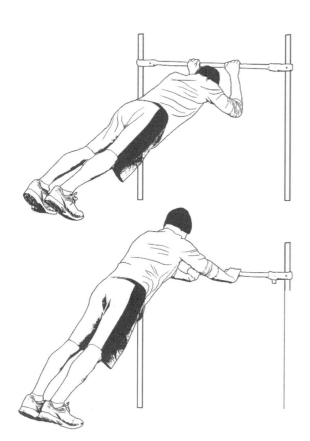

Elbow Press-up

- Position your body over a low bar, with your body straight and toes on the ground.
- Let your elbows bend to lower your head to the bar.
- Straighten your arms to bring yourself back to the starting point.

Pull-up

- Use an overhand grip to hang from a high bar.
- Activate your arms and back muscles to pull your chest to the bar.
- Make sure your chin clears the bar, and then lower yourself back down.
- *Variation:* Use a swinging, or kipping, motion to pull yourself up and down more rapidly.

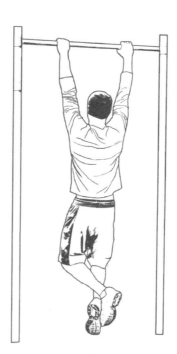

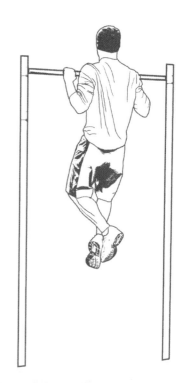

Chin-up

- Hold onto a high bar with an underhand grip, palms toward your face.
- Pull your chest to the bar in one smooth motion.
- Lower yourself back down.
- *Variation:* Try to hold a bent-arm hang for as long as you can.

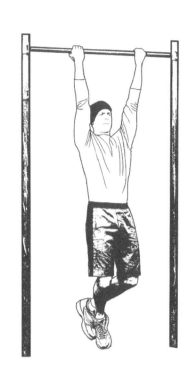 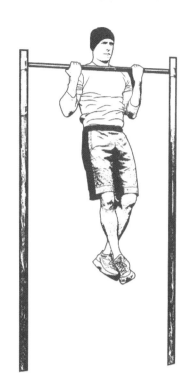

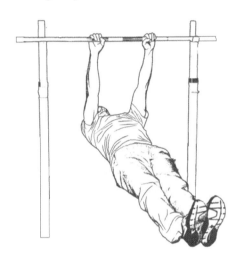

Horizontal Pull-up

- Hang from the underside of a low bar with your feet on the ground.
- Stay tight through your lower body and use your arms to pull your chest to the bar.
- Lower back down to the starting position.
- *Make it harder:* Elevate your feet on a stability ball or bench.

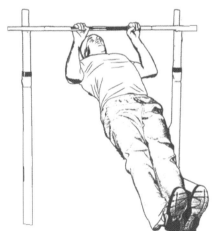

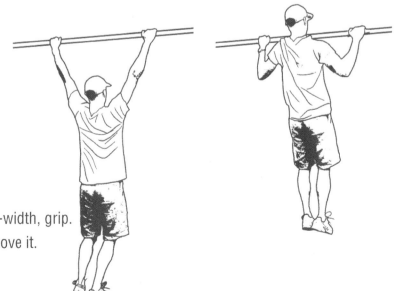

Wide Grip Pull-up

- Hold a high bar with a wide, double shoulder-width, grip.
- Pull your chest to the bar, lifting your chin above it.
- Lower yourself back to the starting position.

Commando Pull-up

- Position yourself sideways under a bar and grab it with a narrow mixed-grip, with each hand grabbing the opposite side of the bar.
- Pull one shoulder to the bar, and then lower to the bottom.
- Switch which side of the bar you bring your head to on each repetition.

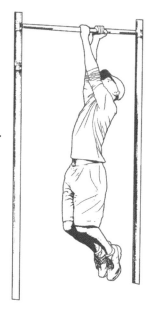 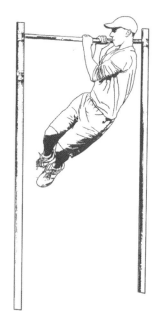

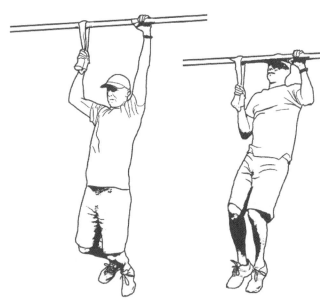

Uneven Pull-up

- Loop a towel or rope around a high bar.
- Grab the bar with one hand and the towel with your other hand.
- Pull yourself up to the bar as high as you can, then return to the bottom.

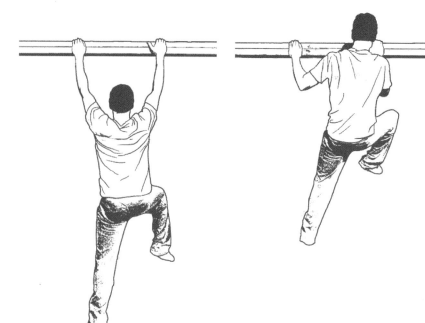

Spiderman Pull-up

- Hold onto a high bar with a basic pull-up grip.
- Lift one knee up to your trunk.
- Keep your knee elevated and pull yourself toward the bar, moving on a diagonal to same side as the raised leg.

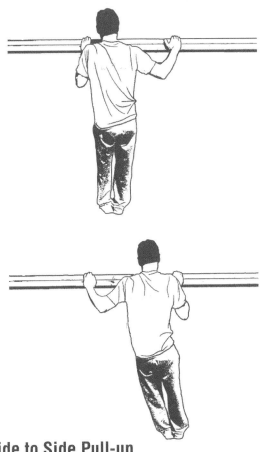

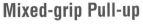

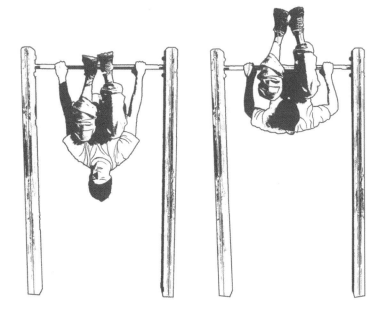

Side to Side Pull-up

- Pull your chest up to a high bar.
- Keep yourself close to the bar and move sideways from one hand to the other.
- Return to the bottom and repeat.

Upside-down Pull-up

- Hang upside-down from a pull-up bar with your knees bent.
- Use your arms to pull yourself upward.
- Touch your bottom to the bar then lower back down.

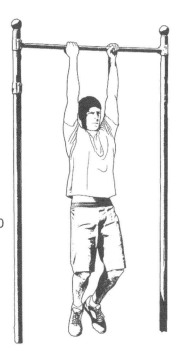

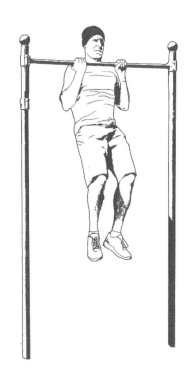

Mixed-grip Pull-up

- Grab a high bar with a mixed-grip, one palm to your face and the other facing away from you.
- Pull your chest to the bar then lower yourself slowly.

Wrist-grip Pull-up

- Grab a pull-up bar with one hand, using your other hand to support that wrist.
- Pull yourself to the bar with the one hand while assisting with your free arm.

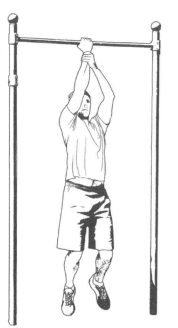
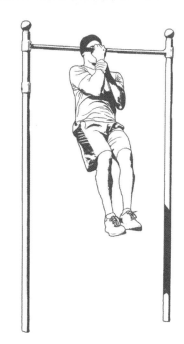

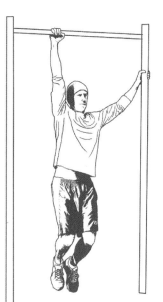
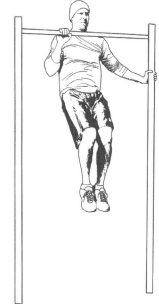

Split Arm Pull-up

- Hang under a pull-up bar with one hand on the bar and the other holding onto the vertical support.
- Pull yourself to the bar with your top hand and with a little assistance from the side hand.

Single Arm Pull-up

- Hang under a pull-up bar using just one hand.
- Tighten your entire body and pull yourself to the bar using the single arm.
- Place your free arm across your body for extra stability during the motion (not shown in the picture).

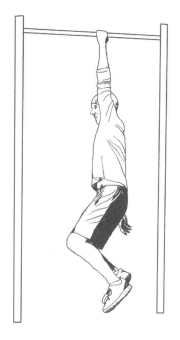
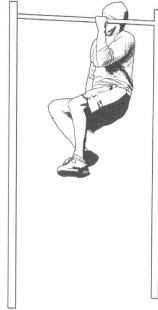

"L" Pull-up

- Hang from a pull-up bar with normal hand placement.
- Raise both legs to be horizontal with the ground in an "L" position.
- Keep your legs elevated and perform the basic Pull-up motion.

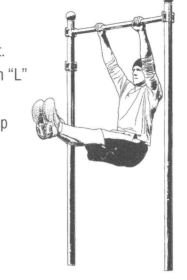
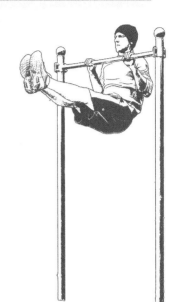

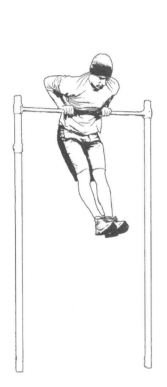
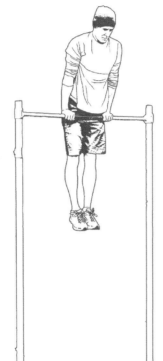

Single Bar Dip

- Position yourself above a high bar with your arms locked in extension.
- Allow your elbows to bend and lower your chest to the bar.
- Keep your weight forward and press yourself back to full extension over the bar.

Muscle-up

- Hang underneath a high bar as if you were going to do a pull-up.
- Pull yourself explosively upward to the bar, bringing your head and chest well above it.
- Immediately roll your shoulders forward to shift your weight into your palms.
- Push downward onto the bar, raising yourself upward until your arms are fully extended.

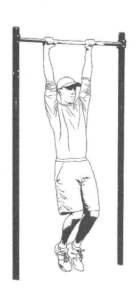
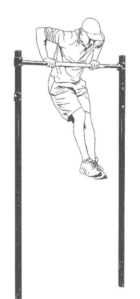
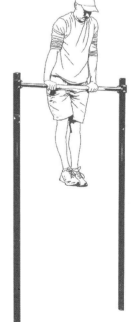

Reverse Dip

- Position yourself above a bar with your pelvis in front of the bar and your hands behind you.
- Grasp the bar with a palms facing forward grip.
- Stay tight through your trunk and allow your arms to bend, lowering your body downward.
- Try not to swing too far under the bar.
- Press through your arms to return to the starting position.

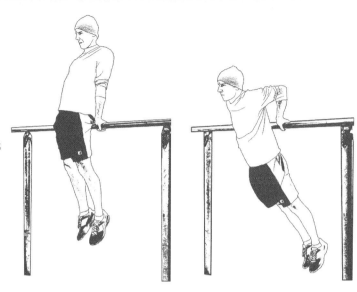

Ice Cream Maker

- Use a regular Pull-up grip and bring your chest up to a high bar.
- Extend your elbows while simultaneously dropping your trunk backward and lifting your legs to horizontal.
- Stay tight through your entire body to maintain a line from your head to feet.
- Reverse the movement, bending your arms to bring your chest back to the bar.

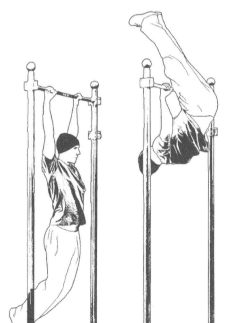

Pull-over

- Hang underneath a high bar as if you were going to do a pull-up.
- Stay tight through your trunk and pull your hips forward and up to the bar.
- Keep your hips moving up and over the bar until you are completely above it with your arms extended.

Tuck Front Lever

- Hang under a high bar with a basic pull-up grip.
- Rock backward until your body is horizontal with the ground while pulling your knees tightly into your chest.
- Keep your head level with your pelvis and try to hold the position as long as you can.
- *Make it harder*: Open up your tuck position, moving to a straddle and then full lower body extension.

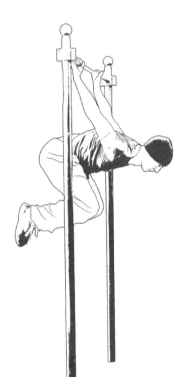

Tuck Back Lever

- Hang under a high bar with a chin-up grip.
- Pull your knees up to your chest while rolling backward through your shoulders.
- Keep moving backward and upside-down, until you have come to the point where your chest is horizontal with the ground.
- Try to keep your head level with your pelvis and hold for as long as you can.
- *Make it harder*: Open your tuck to extend your legs behind you.

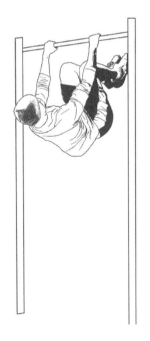
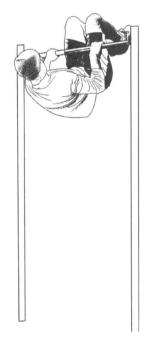

Truck Front Lever Pull-up

- Hang under a high bar and drop your chest backward to assume the Tuck Front Lever position.
- Maintain your body horizontal and use your arms to pull yourself to the bar.
- Return to starting position still in a Tuck Front Lever.
- *Make it harder*: Extend your legs forward into a full front lever.

L-sit

- Sit on the floor with your legs extended and hands placed on the ground, forward of your hips.
- Tighten your trunk and legs while pressing your hands into the ground and lifting your body from the floor.
- Hold the elevated position for as long as you can.

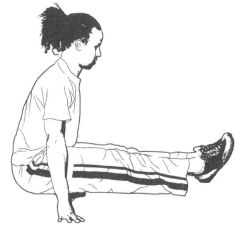

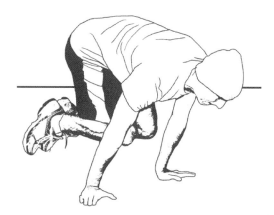

Tuck Planche

- Kneel on the floor and place your hands on the ground under your shoulders.
- Shift your weight forward onto your hands and tighten your lower body into a tuck.
- Pull your feet off the floor and hold the elevated tuck for as long as possible.

Parallette Tuck Hold

- Position yourself over parallettes with your hands directly beneath your shoulders and your chest vertical.
- Tighten your lower body, lifting your feet off the floor into a tuck.
- Stay tight in the tuck and hold the position for as long as possible.

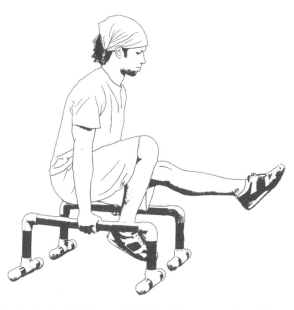

Parallette Single Leg L-sit

- Position yourself over parallettes with both legs extended in front of you.
- Keep your arms and legs locked in extension, then lift your feet from the floor until they are parallel with the ground.
- Stay tight in your lower body and hold the position for as long as possible.

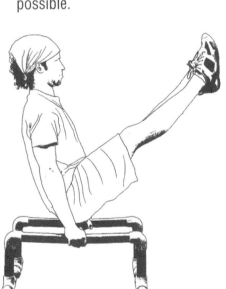

Parallettte L-sit

- Position yourself over parallettes with both legs extended in front of you.
- Keep your arms and legs locked in extension, then lift your feet from the floor until they are parallel with the ground.
- Stay tight in your lower body and hold the position for as long as possible.

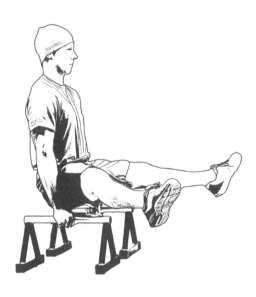

Parallette Straddle L-sit

- Assume an L-sit position above parallettes as previously described.
- Spread your legs apart into a straddle position.
- Stay tight in your lower body and hold the position for as long as possible.

Parallette V-sit

- Begin as if you were going to perform the Parallette L-sit just described.
- Keep raising your feet off the ground until they are at least even with your shoulders.
- Stay tight through your lower body and hold the position for as long as possible.

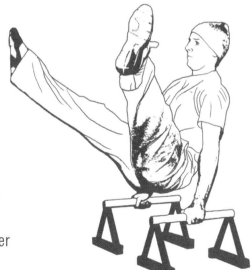

Parallette Straddle V-sit

- Begin as if you were going to perform a Parallette V-sit, except spread your legs wide.
- Shift your weight into your hands and lift your legs from the floor, with your feet spread apart.
- Try to drive your hips as far forward as you can without falling over backward.

Parallette Dip

- Place yourself over parallettes with your feet in front of you, resting on a medicine ball or other elevated surface.
- Bend your elbows to lower your hips to the floor.
- Press your arms back into extension to lift your body back to the starting position.

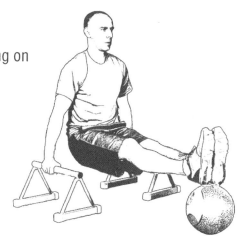

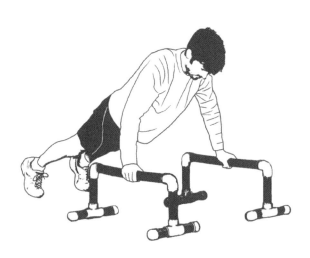

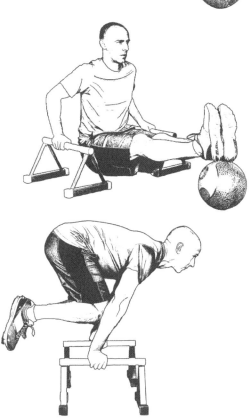

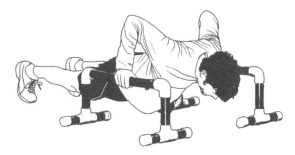

Parallette Push-up

- Position your trunk over parallettes with your hands beneath your shoulders.
- Let your arms bend to bring your chest to your hands.
- Stay tight through your lower body and press your chest upward again.

Parallette Tuck Planche

- Crouch on the ground with your hands placed on parallettes.
- Shift your weight forward onto your hands while lifting your feet off the ground.
- Pull your knees into a tuck and keep your shoulders level with your hips.
- *Make it harder*: Open up the tuck, extending your legs behind you.

Parallette Handstand Push-up

- Place parallettes next to a wall and kick up to a handstand.
- Stay tight in your trunk and lower your head to the floor, between your hands.
- Press yourself upward until your arms are fully extended.
- *Make it harder:* Try it free standing, away from a wall!

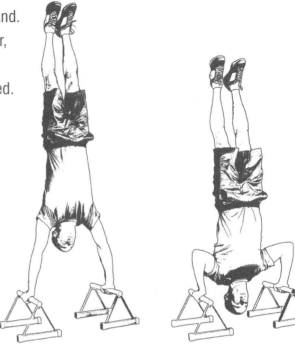

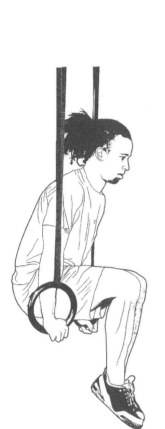

Ring Tuck Hold

- Elevate your body above gymnastics rings with your arms fully extended.
- Lift your knees upward into a tuck position.
- Squeeze the rings inward and hold the tuck for as long as possible.

Ring L-sit

- Elevate your body above gymnastics rings with your arms fully extended.
- Lift your legs in front of you, keeping them completely straight.
- Stay tight across your lower body and hold the position for as long as possible.

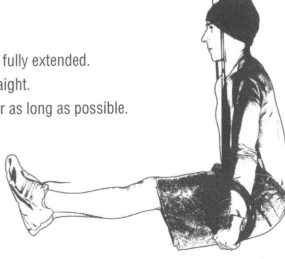

Ring Dip

- Elevate your body above gymnastics rings with your arms fully extended.
- Bend your elbows to lower your chest to your hands.
- Squeeze the rings inward and press yourself back up to the starting position.

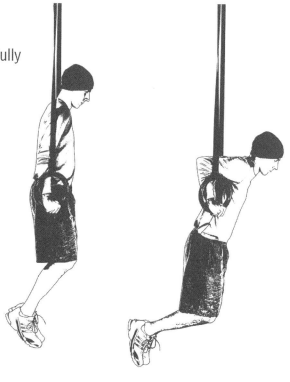

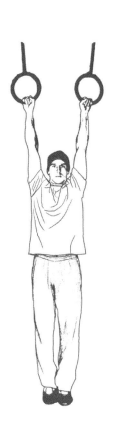

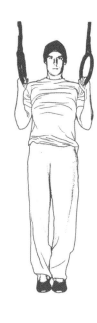

Ring Pull-up

- Hang underneath rings with your arms relaxed in full extension.
- Pull your chest to the rings, bringing your chin above your hands.
- Lower yourself back to the starting position.

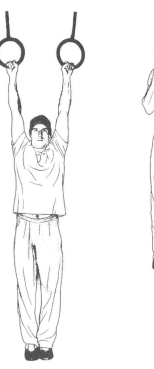

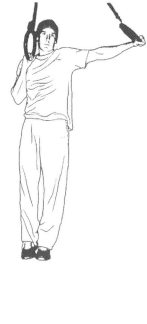

Archer Pull-up

- Start in the Ring Pull-up position just described.
- As you pull your chest up to the rings, extend one arm outward to the side as if you were drawing a bow.
- Lower back to the starting position, allowing your hand to return to the center.

Ring Muscle-up

- Hang under rings as if you were about to perform a pull-up.
- Explode upward, pulling your chest above your hands.
- Roll your shoulders forward, squeeze the rings inward, and press your arms into full extension.

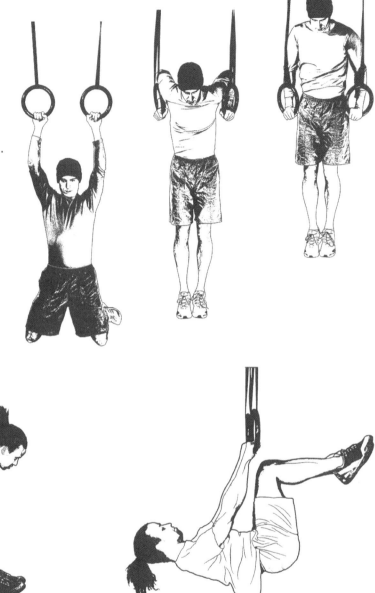

Skin the Cat

- Hang beneath rings and begin pulling your hips upward.
- Raise your pelvis until you are upside-down and keep rolling backward through your shoulders.
- Let your feet descend backward as far as you comfortably can and hang in this position for a few moments.
- Reverse the movement and roll back between your shoulders until you are upside-down again.

Ring Tuck Front Lever

- Hang beneath rings and pull your knees into a tuck position.
- Keep raising your hips as you let your trunk rock backward.
- Stop your motion once your back is horizontal and your head is level with your pelvis. Hold the position for as long as you can.
- *Make it harder:* Open your tuck into a straddle or until your legs are fully extended.

Ring Bicep Curl

- Hang beneath a low pair of rings with your legs extended and heels on the ground.
- Keep your elbows tucked to your sides and bend your arms, bringing your chin to the rings.
- Isolate the motion to your elbows for an effective body-weight bicep curl.

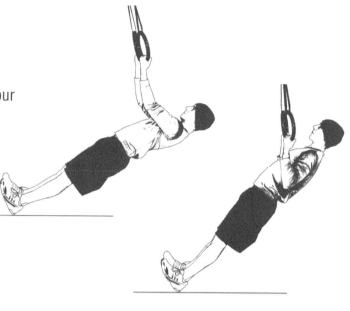

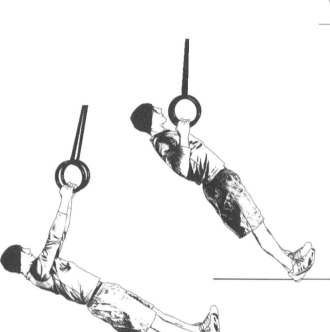

Ring Row

- Hang beneath a pair of low rings with your legs extended and heels on the ground.
- Let your elbows flare outward and pull your chest to the rings.
- Squeeze your shoulder blades together as a great body-weight exercise for your back.
- *Variation:* Elevate your feet on a bench or stability ball.

Ring Push-up

- Position your body over rings that are 6 to 18 inches above the ground.
- Place your feet on the ground behind you, and then bend your arms to lower your chest to your hands.
- Squeeze the rings inward and press yourself upward to the starting position.
- *Make it harder:* Elevate your feet on a bench or stability ball.

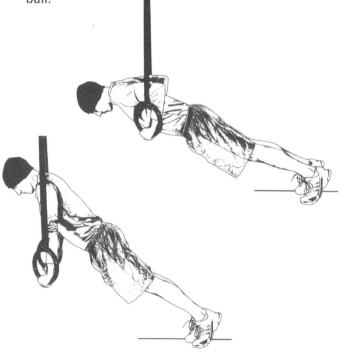

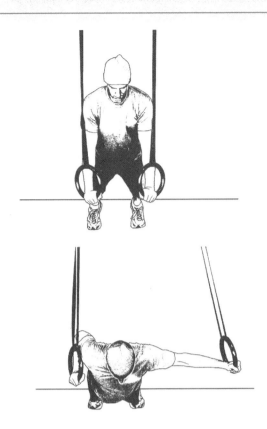

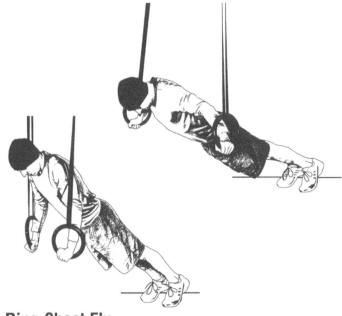

Ring Chest Fly

- Start in the same position as the Ring Push-up.
- Carefully let your arms spread apart, so that you lower your chest toward the floor.
- Stay tight across your upper body and squeeze the rings, bringing your hands back together.

Archer Push-up

- Start in the same position as the Ring Push-up previously described.
- Lower your trunk toward the floor while keeping one hand under your chest and driving the other hand away from your body.
- Squeeze the rings underneath you as you press back to the starting position.

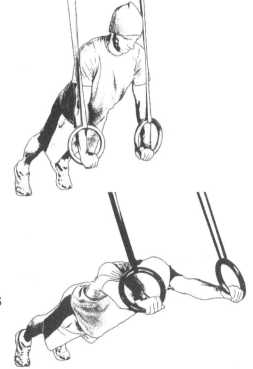

Ring Roll-out

- Start in the same position as the Ring Push-up.
- Stay tight in your trunk and shoulders and press the rings forward and away from your body.
- Allow your trunk to lower toward the floor and then pull the rings back underneath you to return to the starting position.

Chapter 9

"Without a sturdy core, your ability to generate power from your limbs is hampered and you end up a less efficient beast."

Midriff Maintenance

Strong arms let you hang, throw, row, and push things. Strong legs let you run, jump, bike, and skate. The gray matter between your ears coordinates it all, giving guidance to how you steer your body. What about your often neglected trunk region? Without a sturdy core, your ability to generate power from your limbs is hampered and you end up a less efficient beast.

Think about it this way: Most athletic skills involve compound movements, demanding a fair amount of cooperation between your upper and lower body. If your middle section is weak, translating the forces generated by your hips into your shoulders is severely impaired.

A boxer's punch is a perfect example. A subtle shift in the hips initiates a rotation of the trunk that gives extra oomph to the shoulders, yielding a whip-like punch. Any weakness in the midsection leads to a loss of upper-body force.

How does your middle section perform this critical bridging between your upper and lower body? There are five key functions that best describe the skeletal-muscle action of your core:

- **Movement constraint:** Getting rid of excess movement in your trunk allows the smooth translation of lower to upper body force. The plank—and all of its derivatives—is the most tried-and-true method for achieving this function.

- **Trunk flexion:** Flexing your spine to bring your head and pelvis closer together is a fundamental motion, used any time you jump or get up from a reclined position. Exercises like crunches, sit-ups, and leg lifts are the best ways to strengthen this movement.

- **Trunk extension:** Bringing the back of your head toward your butt might not seem like it's that important of a motion, but it is. Weak trunk extension makes swimming or doing a back flip downright impossible.

- **Trunk rotation:** Anytime you perform a spinning movement, whether it's a 360 on a snowboard or a tornado kick in karate, the spin is initiated with trunk rotation. Your abdomen contracts to rotate your upper body, and the force is then translating through your spine to move your lower body. Having a strong abdomen allows you to spin more effectively.

- **Trunk side bending:** At first thought, collapsing your ribcage toward your pelvis might not seem like it's used all that often in athletic skills. But consider trying to do a cartwheel or a side-flip without allowing your trunk to flex laterally. Those are skills unique to acrobatics, but you get the picture: Bending sideways is an essential movement.

It's valuable to mention that out of those five muscle actions of your abdominal region, a sixth skill is derived: diagonal, multi-planar movement. By pairing extension or flexion with rotation or side bending, you begin to move in a more complex pattern. Complexity is the calling card of life and so with athletic ability.

There are over 100 exercises in this chapter to address each of the movement classes listed above. Don't get stagnant with just a few variations of crunches and planks. Draw heavily from each category and you'll naturally sculpt your trunk into a muscular powerhouse, capable of propelling you to athletic feats never before imagined.

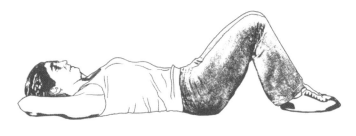

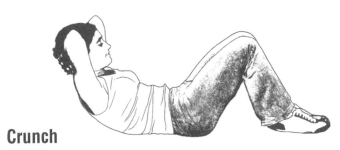

Crunch

- Lie on the ground with your knees bent, feet flat on the floor, and hands behind your head.
- Tighten your abdominal muscles to lift your head and chest off the floor.
- Lift high enough to raise your shoulder blades from the ground, and then return to the starting position.

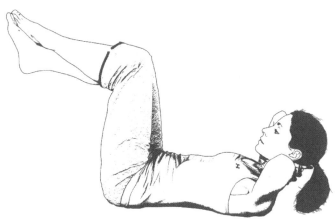

Raised Knee Crunch

- Perform the Crunch motion, with your feet lifted off the floor.
- Try to maintain your ankles level with your knees as you lift your torso.

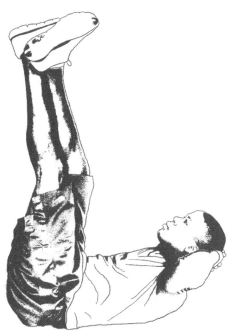

Raised Leg Crunch

- Perform a Crunch with your legs raised straight to the ceiling.
- Keep your ankles crossed for greater stability.

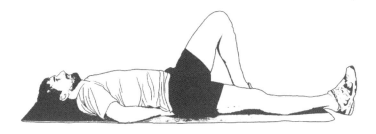

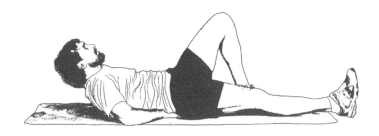

Modified Crunch

- Lie on the floor with one leg straight and the other bent with the foot flat on the ground.
- Place your hands under your low back or behind your head.
- Tighten your abdominal muscles to lift your upper torso off the ground, as with a Crunch.

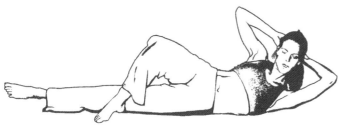

Oblique Crunch

- Lie on one side of your body, using your top leg to provide balance.
- Place your hands behind your head.
- Activate your lateral trunk muscles and lift your head and shoulders off the floor.

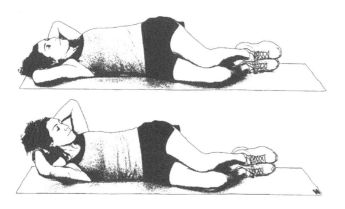

Rotated Crunch

- Lie on the ground with your shoulders flat on the floor and your lower body rotated 90 degrees to one side.
- Place your hands behind your head and perform the Crunch motion from this position.

Twisting Crunch

- Start in the Crunch position, with your knees bent and hands behind your head.
- As you lift your shoulders from the floor drive one elbow toward the opposite knee, making your upper body to twist.
- Alternate sides on each repetition.

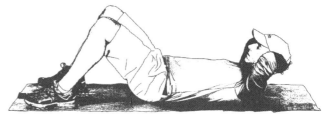

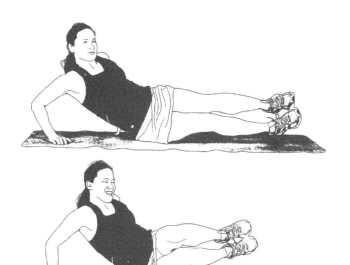

Semi-reclined Side Crunch

- Use your arms to support yourself in a semi-reclined position on one hip.
- Keeping your feet off the floor, pull them into your body in a reverse crunching motion.

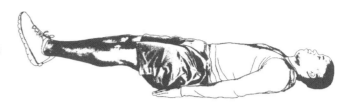

Reverse Crunch

- Lie on the ground with your hands under your hips and feet off the floor.
- Tighten your abdominal muscles and pull your knees to your chest in a reverse crunching motion.

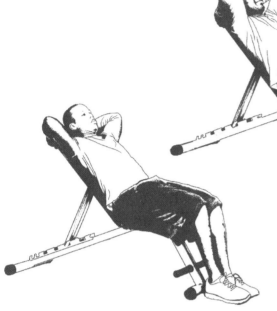

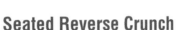

Seated Reverse Crunch

- Sit on an angled weight bench, grabbing the top of the bench behind your head to keep from slipping down.
- Pull your knees to your chest in a reverse crunching motion.

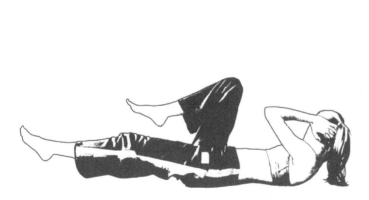

Bicycle Crunch

- Lie on the ground with both feet off the floor and your hands behind your head.
- Lift one knee to your chest and drive your opposite elbow towards it in a twisting crunch motion.
- Alternate sides on each repetition.

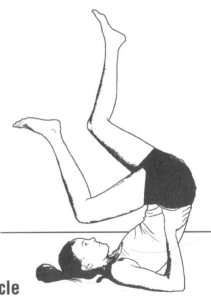

Inverted Bicycle

- Use your hands on your trunk to support yourself in a semi-inverted position.
- Kick your legs to the ceiling one at a time in a bicycling motion.

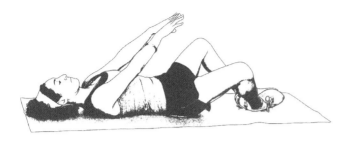

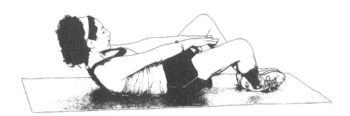

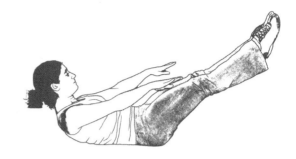

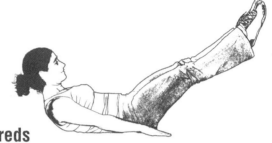

Frog Leg Crunch

- Lie on the floor with your knees bent and thighs spread apart.
- Lift your upper trunk off the ground and reach your hands between your legs.

Hundreds

- Lie on the floor with your legs held off the ground on a 45-degree angle.
- Lift your head and shoulders off the ground, with your arms extended along your torso.
- Maintain this position while slowly pumping your arms up and down.

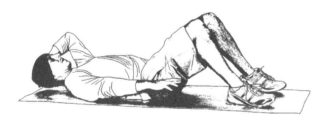

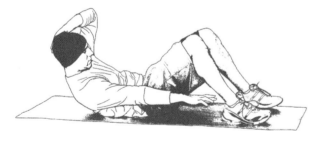

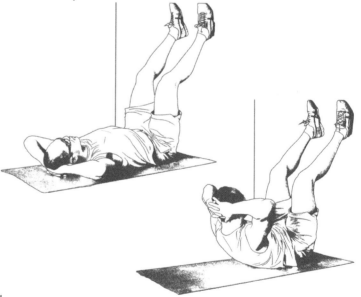

Fish Hook Crunch

- Lie on the floor with your knees bent, with one hand behind your head, and the other hand extended along your torso.
- Lift your upper trunk from the ground, while reaching your free hand toward your foot.

Feet on Wall Crunch

- Lie on the floor with your feet elevated and resting against a wall.
- Keep your hands behind your head and lift your torso in a Crunch.

Toe Touch Crunch

- Lie on the floor with your legs held straight to the ceiling.
- Extend your arms above your chest and then perform a crunch, reaching your fingers to your toes.

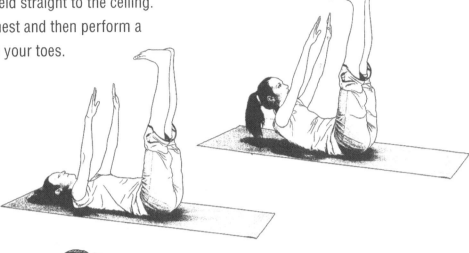

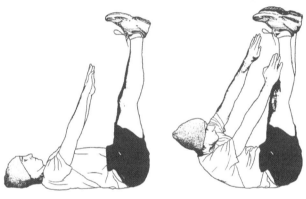

Twisting Toe Touch

- Lie on the ground with your legs held straight to the ceiling.
- Extend your arms above your chest and perform a crunch, reaching your fingers to the outer part of one leg.
- Alternate the side you reach toward on each repetition.

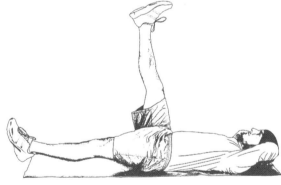

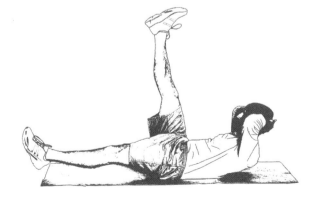

Split Leg Crunch

- Lie on the floor with one leg held to the ceiling and the other lifted a few inches off the ground.
- Place your hands behind your head and lift your chest in a Crunch motion.
- *Variation:* Hold your arms straight above your chest and reach for your raised leg on each repetition.

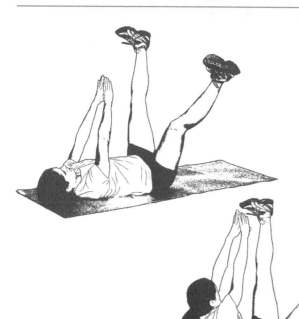

"V" Spread Toe Touch

- Lie on the floor with your legs held above you, split apart in a "V" formation.
- Hold your arms above your chest and then perform a crunch, reaching your hands toward one of your feet.
- Alternate which leg you reach to, on each repetition.

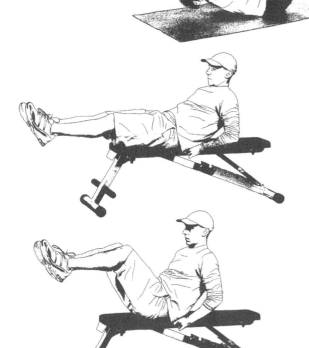

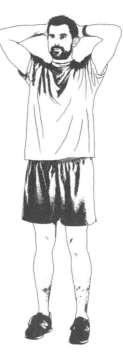

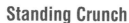

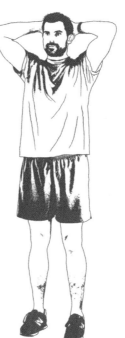

Rowing Crunch

- Use your hands to support yourself in a semi-reclined position.
- Keep your chest and feet lifted off the ground or bench.
- Pull your knees into your chest and then extend them outward again.

Standing Crunch

- Stand with your hands placed behind your head.
- Lift one knee and lower the opposite elbow toward it in a twisting motion.
- March back and forth, alternating sides on each repetition.

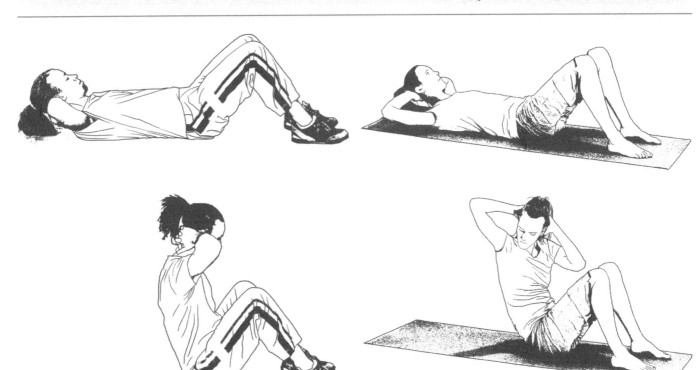

Sit-up

- Lie on the floor with your knees bent and hands placed behind your head.
- Tighten your trunk and hips to lift your torso completely off the floor.
- Continue lifting until your chest is near your thighs.

Negative Sit-up

- Sit on the ground with your knees bent and chest positioned close to your thighs.
- Slowly lower backward, curling your spine to the ground.
- Stop before your shoulders touch the ground and then reverse direction back to the starting position.

Alternating Sit-up

- Lie on the floor with your knees bent and hands placed behind your head.
- Lift your entire trunk off the ground and reach one elbow to your opposite knee.
- Alternate sides on each repetition.

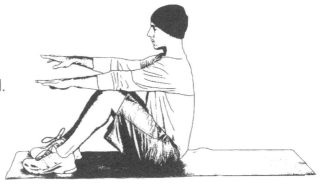

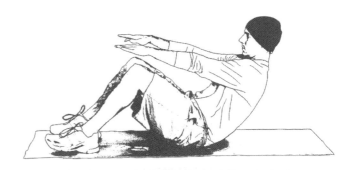

Modified Sit-up

- Lie on the ground with one knee bent and the other leg held off the floor.
- Place your hands behind your head and perform a Sit-up, bringing your chest to your thigh.
- Keep your free leg off the ground throughout the entire movement.

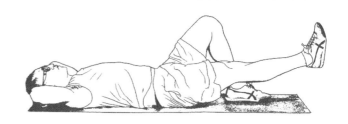

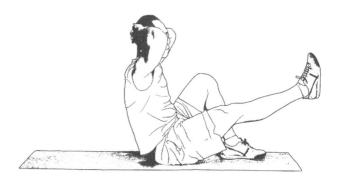

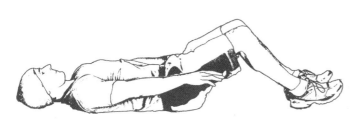

Knee Grab Sit-up

- Lie on the floor in a Sit-up position.
- Tighten your abdominal muscles and lift your trunk and feet off the floor.
- Grab your knees before returning to the ground.

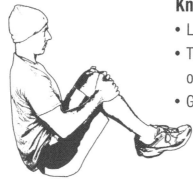

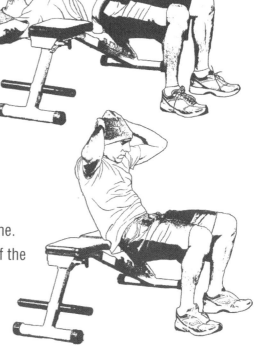

Bench Sit-up

- Squat perpendicular to a weight bench with your low back supported against its cushion.
- Allow your trunk to extend over the bench, arching your spine.
- Tighten your abdominal muscles to lift your chest up and off the bench in a Sit-up motion.

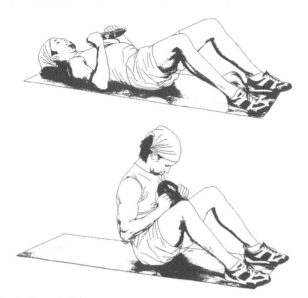

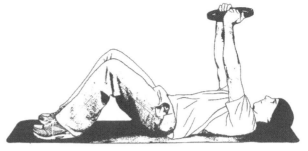

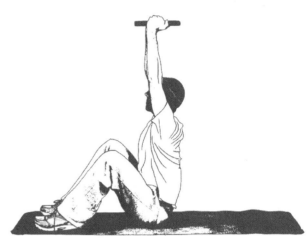

Weighted Sit-up

- Get on the floor in a Sit-up position, holding a weight plate at your chest.
- Perform a Sit-up, holding the weight plate as extra resistance.
- *Variation:* Hold a medicine ball, dumbbell, or kettlebell.

Overhead Weighted Sit-up

- Lie on the floor with your knees bent while holding a weight plate above your chest with arms extended.
- Perform a Sit-up, and push the weight plate toward the ceiling.
- Keep your arms straight throughout the movement.

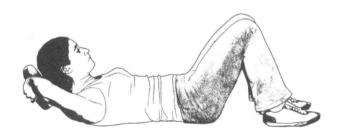

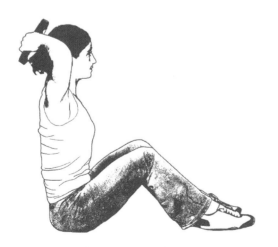

Behind the Head Weighted Sit-up

- Lie on the floor with your knees bent, while holding a weight plate behind your head.
- Keep the weight behind your head as you perform a Sit-up movement.

Roll-up

- Lie on the floor with your legs fully extended and arms elongated beyond your head.
- Roll your torso off the ground, reaching forward with your arms.
- Keep reaching forward with your legs on the floor and finish in an upright sitting position.

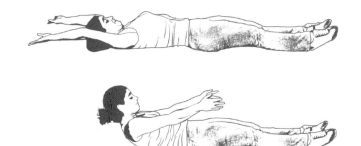

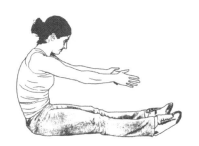

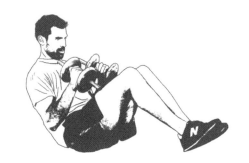

Butterfly Sit-up

- Lie on the floor with your arms spread wide and legs held a few inches from the ground.
- Bring your hands together while lifting your chest and pulling your knees upward.
- Open your arms and legs and lower back to the floor.
- *Make it harder:* Hold two dumbbells for extra resistance.

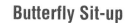

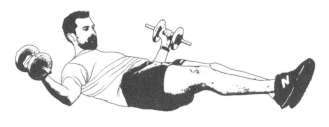

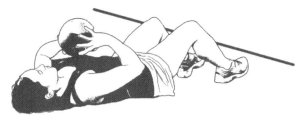

Sit-up Wall Ball

- Lie on the floor with your knees bent and feet placed close to a wall.
- Hold a medicine ball at your chest.
- Complete a Sit-up while simultaneously throwing the ball to the wall.
- Catch the ball and return to the floor gently.

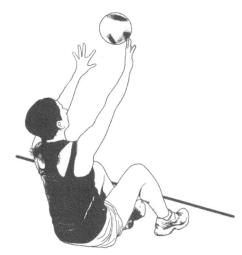

Full Arc Sit-up

- Sit on a pair of parallel bars with your feet hooked under one bar and your hips supported on the other bar.
- Lower your head and trunk backward to the ground behind you.
- Tighten your abdominal muscles and perform a full arc sit-up, raising your chest back up to the starting position.
- *Make it harder:* Keep your arms extended above your head.

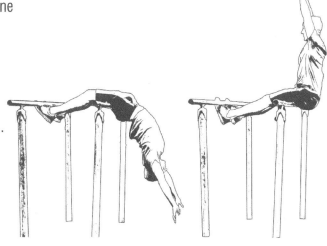

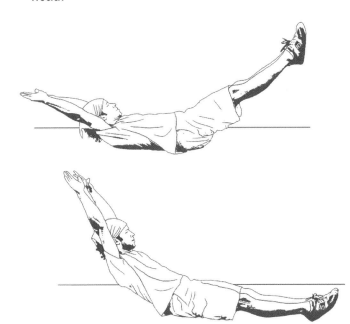

Hollow Rock

- Lie on the floor with your arms and legs extended off the ground.
- Flatten your spine to the floor by tightening your belly.
- Begin rocking back and forth, alternately touching your feet and hands to the ground.
- *Variation:* Simply holding the "hollow" position with your arms and legs off the floor can be an effective core strength exercise.

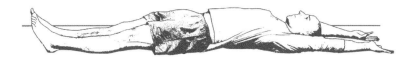

V-up

- Lie on the floor with your legs fully extended and your arms elongated beyond your head.
- Tighten your core and hinge at your waist, lifting your legs and reaching forward with your arms.
- Try to touch your fingers to your feet, then return to the starting position.

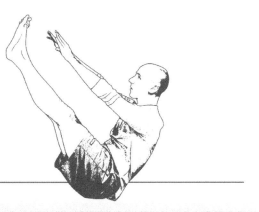

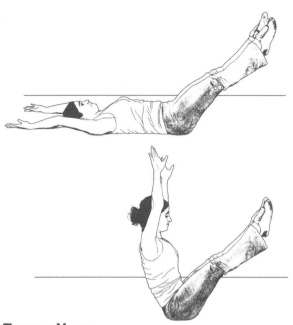

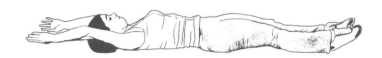

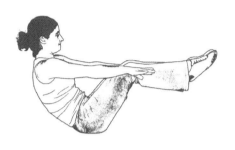

Teaser V-up

- Lie on the floor with your arms extended and legs lifted off the floor at a 45-degree angle.
- Tighten your abdominal muscles and lift your chest off the ground, reaching your hands upward.

Tuck-up

- Lie on the floor with your legs fully extended and your arms elongated beyond your head.
- Pull your knees inward and lift your upper body off the ground into a tucked position.

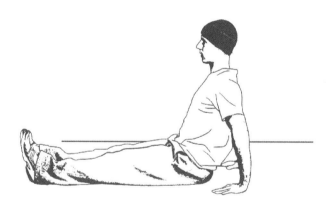

Double Leg Raise

- Sit on the floor with your legs extended and hands placed by your hips.
- Tighten your core and lift both legs off the ground as high as you can.
- *Make it harder:* Place your hands farther forward along your thighs, forcing more trunk compression.

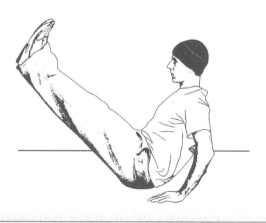

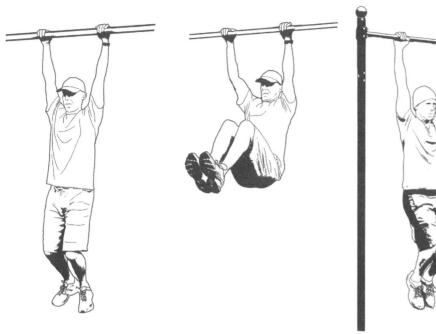

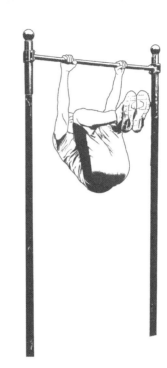

Hanging Knee Raise

- Hang from a high bar, using a normal Pull-up grip.
- Lift both knees to your chest, keeping your feet together.

Knee to Elbows

- Start in the same position as the Hanging Knee Raise.
- Lift your knees all the way until they touch your elbows.

Toes to Bar

- Hang from a high bar, using a normal Pull-up grip.
- Keep your legs straight and lift both feet all the way to the bar, trying not to drop your chest too far backward.
- Lower your legs with smooth control.

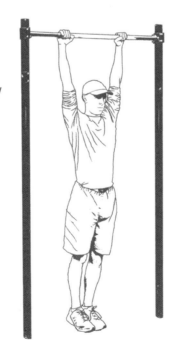

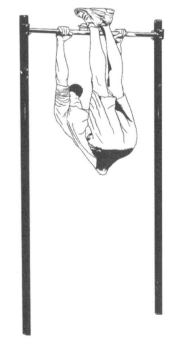

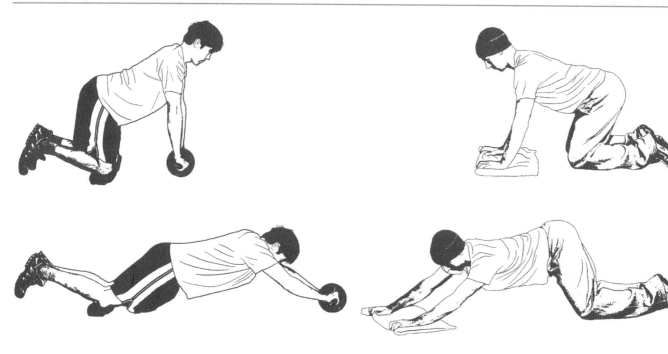

Ab Roller

- Kneel on the floor, holding a small ab roller on the ground under your shoulders.
- Push the roller forward along the ground, dropping your torso to horizontal.
- Pull the roller back to your knees to return to the starting position.
- *Variation:* If you don't have an ab wheel, use a dumbbell or weight plate with a small dowel.

Floor Scrub

- Kneel on the floor with your hands placed on a towel underneath your shoulders.
- Reach forward as far as you can, then pull back to the starting position.
- *Make it harder:* Vary your angle of motion off to each side.

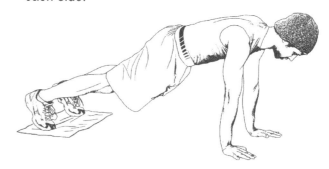

Towel Drag

- Get on the floor in a Push-up position with your feet placed on a towel.
- Pull your feet inward to your hands, into a pike position.
- Push the towel backward to return to the beginning.

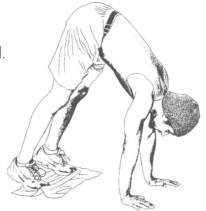

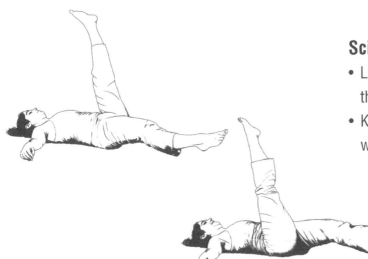

Scissors

- Lie on the floor with one foot lifted to the ceiling and the other hovering above the floor.
- Keep your abdomen tight and lower the top leg while lifting the bottom leg, switching their position.

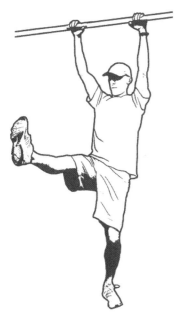
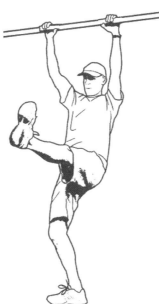

Hanging Leg Scissors

- Hang from a high bar, using a normal Pull-up grip.
- Lift one leg to the horizontal, and then lower it while simultaneously lifting the other leg.
- Keep lifting your legs in a scissoring motion.

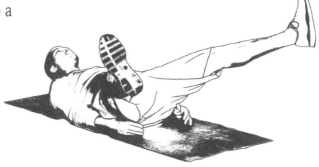

Horizontal Scissors

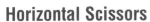

- Lie on the floor with your feet held a few inches off the ground.
- Tighten your core and then open and close your legs in a scissoring motion.

Flutter Kick

- Lie on the floor with both feet elevated off the ground.
- Stay tight in your abdomen and kick your legs up and down in a compact version of the scissoring motion.

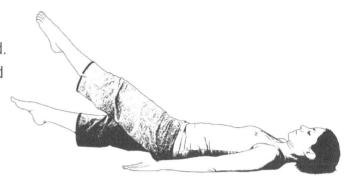

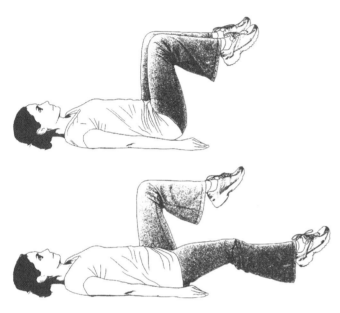

Single Leg Extension

- Lie on the floor with both feet off the ground and your knees positioned over your pelvis.
- Tighten your core and then lower one leg to the ground at a time.
- Alternate which leg you lower on every repetition.

Double Leg Extension

- Lie on the floor with both feet off the ground and your knees positioned over your pelvis.
- Tighten your core and extend both legs down toward the ground.
- Pull your legs back to the starting position before they touch the floor.

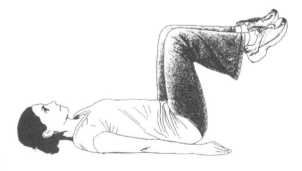

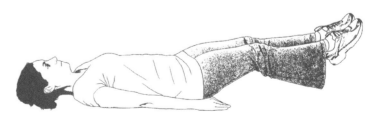

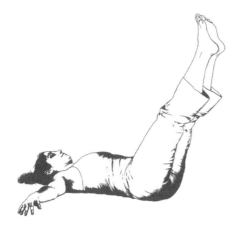

Leg Drop

- Lie on the ground and hold both legs straight above you.
- Tighten your core and lower your legs toward the floor, but don't let them touch down.
- Raise your legs back above your body and repeat.

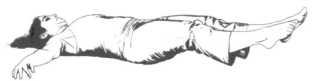

Med Ball Leg Drops

- Lie on the ground and use your feet to hold a medicine ball above your body.
- Tighten your core and lower the ball to the floor.
- Reverse directions before you touch the ground.

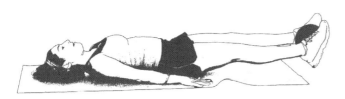

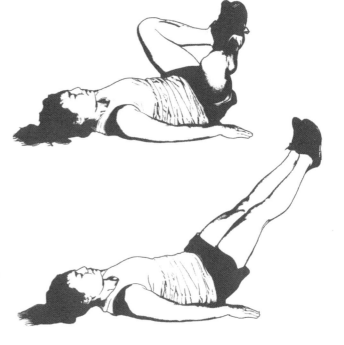

Frog Leg Raise

- Lie on the ground with your feet pulled toward your chest and your knees spread apart.
- Tighten your core and push your feet away from your body at a 45-degree angle.
- Pull your knees back to your torso and repeat.

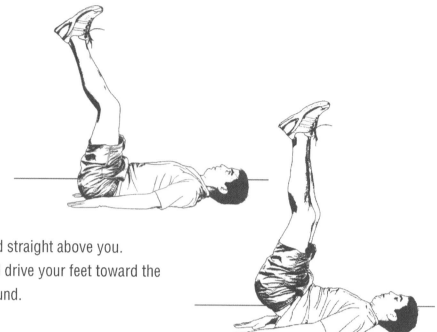

Pelvic Thrust

- Lie on the ground with your legs held straight above you.
- Tighten your abdominal muscles and drive your feet toward the ceiling, lifting your pelvis off the ground.

Twisting Pelvic Thrust

- Lie on the ground with your legs held straight above you.
- Tighten your abdominal muscles and drive your feet to the ceiling while twisting your hips so that your pelvis comes off the ground on an angle.

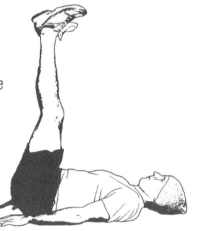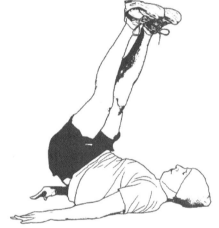

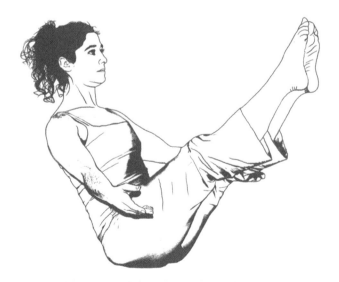

V-sit

- Sit on the ground, balancing on your butt with your legs held straight.
- Point your toes and keep your feet as high off the ground as you can.
- Stay tight through your core and hold for as long as you can.

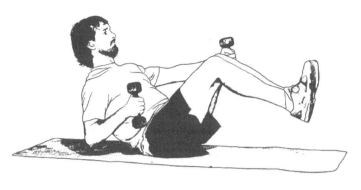

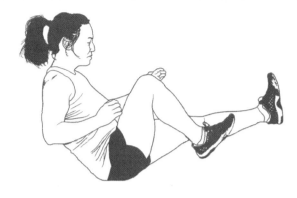

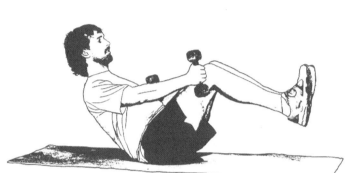

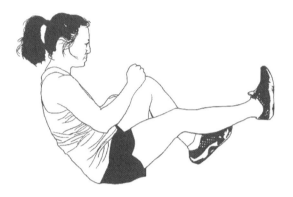

Rowing V-sit

- Sit on the ground, balancing on your butt with your feet held off the ground.
- Stay tight in your core and pump your arms forward and backward in an alternating motion.
- *Make it harder:* Hold a pair of dumbbells.

Sprinting V-sit

- Sit on the ground, balancing on your butt with your legs held off the floor.
- Kick your legs in and out in a running motion.
- Pump your fists up and down, imitating a natural running movement.

Rope Climbing V-sit

- Sit on the ground, balancing on your butt with your legs held off the floor.
- Reach one hand overhead as if you were grabbing a rope.
- Pull your top hand down and raise the other hand up as if you were climbing a rope.
- Move your legs in and out as if they were helping you climb.

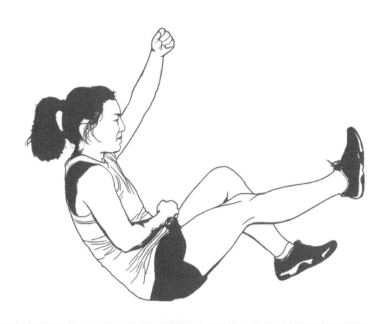

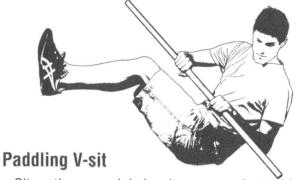

Paddling V-sit

- Sit on the ground, balancing on your butt with your feet elevated.
- Hold a dowel or barbell, and twist your torso side to side as if you were paddling a kayak.

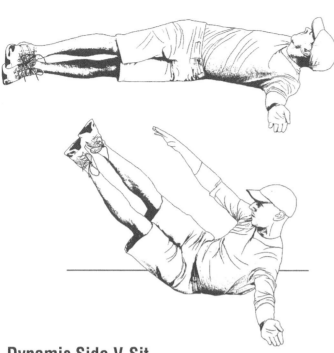

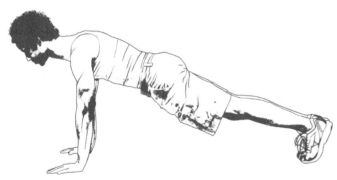

Dynamic Side V-Sit

- Lie on the ground, resting on one side of your body.
- Push through your bottom hand while lifting both legs off the floor.
- Flex as much as you can through your trunk and try to touch your top hand to your toes.

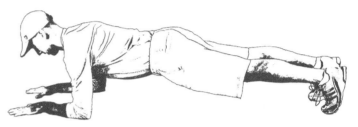

Plank on Elbows

- Place your forearms on the ground, extend your lower body behind you, and balance on your tiptoes.
- Lock your shoulders, maintain a neutral spine position, and stay tight through your core.
- Try to hold the position for as long as you can.

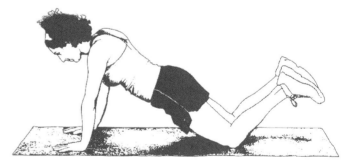

Plank

- Place your hands on the ground, extend your lower body behind you, and balance on your tiptoes.
- Lock your shoulders, maintain a neutral spine position, and stay tight through your core.
- Try to hold the position for as long as you can.

Modified Plank

- Place your hands on the ground, extend your lower body behind you, and balance on your knees.
- Lock your shoulders, maintain a neutral spine position, and stay tight through your core.
- Hold the position for as long as you can.

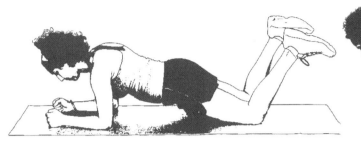

Modified Plank on Elbows

- Place your forearms on the ground and perform the Modified Plank as just described.

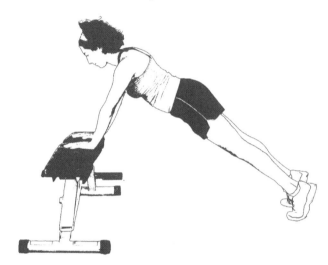

Elevated Plank

- Place your hands on a weight bench and extend your lower body behind you, balancing on your tiptoes.
- Lock your shoulders, maintain a neutral spine position, and stay tight through your core.

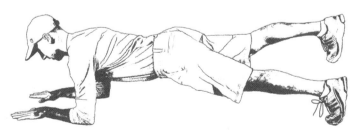

3-point Plank on Elbows

- Place your forearms on the ground and perform the 3-point Plank as just described.

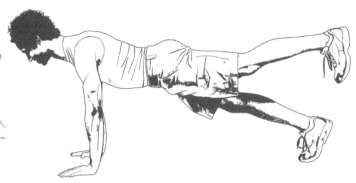

3-point Plank

- Place your hands on the ground, extend your lower body behind you, and balance on one foot.
- Hold your other leg off the ground as high as you can.
- Lock your shoulders, maintain a neutral spine position, and stay tight through your core.

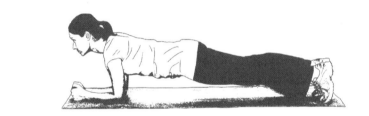

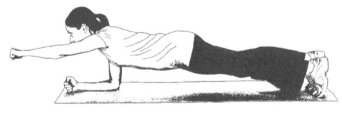

Plank Arm Raise

- Place your forearms on the ground, extend your lower body, and balance on your tiptoes.
- Hold the Plank and lift one arm off the ground as high as you can.
- *Make it harder*: Support yourself on your hands instead of your forearms.

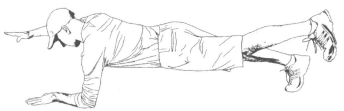
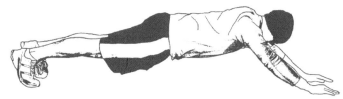

2-point Plank

- Place your forearms on the ground, extend your lower body, and balance on one foot.
- Hold the 3-point Plank and then lift one arm off the ground as high as you can.
- *Make it harder:* Support yourself on your hand instead of your forearm.

Extended Plank

- Place your hands on the ground, positioned above your shoulders and head.
- Extend your lower body behind you and balance on your tiptoes.
- Tighten your shoulders, hips, and core.
- Try to hold your body off the ground for as long as you can.

Dynamic Plank

- Place your forearms on the ground and assume a Plank position.
- Push through your elbows and lift your bottom to the ceiling as high as you can.
- Return to the starting position and repeat.

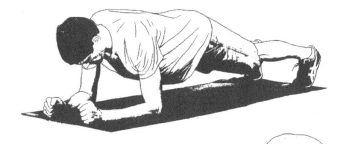

Rotated Plank

- Place your hands on the ground and extend your lower body behind you, rotating your pelvis 90 degrees to one side.
- Stack your feet on top of each other, lock your shoulders, and tighten your core.
- Try to maintain the position for as long as you can.

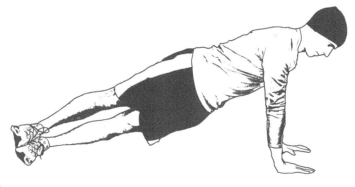

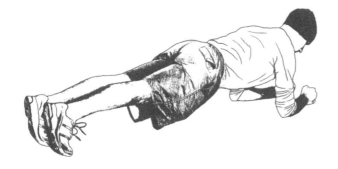

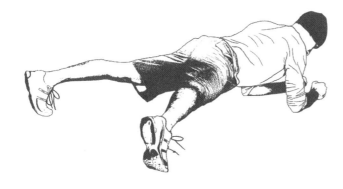

Plank Splits

- Get on the ground in a Plank position, supported on your hands or elbows.
- Tighten your shoulders and abdomen, and then jump your legs wide apart.
- Hop them back together, and then keep moving them apart and together.

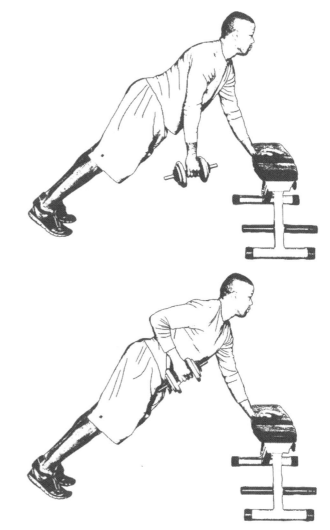

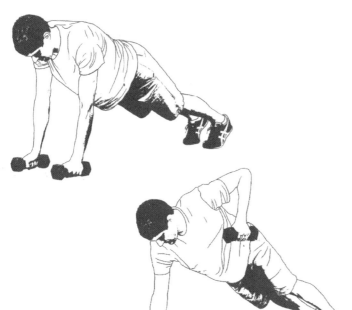

Plank Row

- Support yourself on the ground in a basic Plank position.
- Pull one hand to your chest, lower it to the floor, and then repeat on the other side.
- *Make it harder:* Hold a dumbbell in each hand.

Supported Plank Row

- Place one hand on a weight bench with your lower body extended behind you in a Plank position.
- Hold a dumbbell in your free hand and row it to your chest while staying tight through your hips, abdomen, and opposite shoulder.

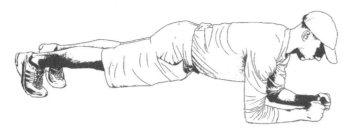

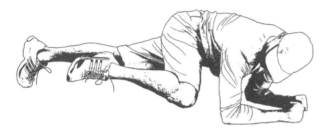

Plank Side Crunch

- Place your forearms on the ground and assume a Plank position.
- Tighten your core and lift one knee up and out to the side.
- Try to bring your knee all the way to your elbow while allowing your body to perform a slight crunch.

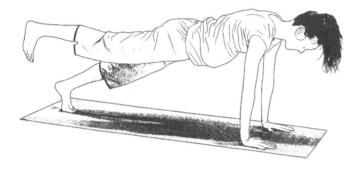

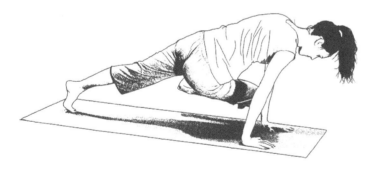

Twisting Plank

- Place your hands on the ground and assume a 3-point Plank with one foot lifted off the floor.
- Drive your free leg up and under you, toward your opposite elbow.

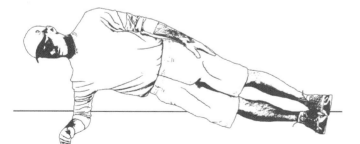

Side Plank on Elbow

- Place one forearm on the ground and balance on your side with your weight between your elbow and outer foot.
- Tighten your shoulder, core, and hips and try to maintain the position for as long as you can.

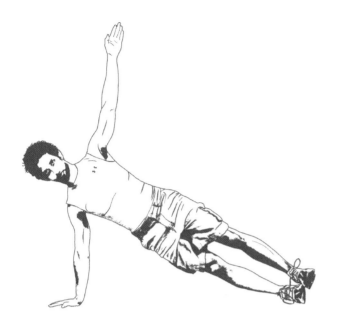

Side Plank

- Place one hand on the floor and stack your feet together so you are balancing between your hand and outer foot.
- Stay tight through your shoulder, trunk, and hips to maintain a straight line through your body.
- Hold your top arm overhead and stay in the position for as long as you can.

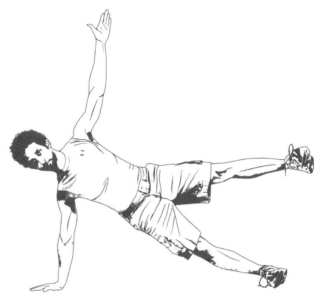

Side Plank & Leg Lift

- Position yourself on the ground in a Side Plank, balanced between one hand and foot.
- Raise your top leg while keeping your foot parallel with the ground.
- Tighten through your shoulders, core, and hips and try to hold the position for as long as possible.

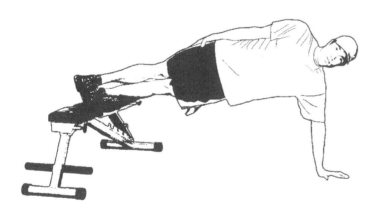

Side Plank - Feet Elevated

- Place one hand on the ground and elevate your feet on a weight bench.
- Hold your body in a Side Plank for as long as you can.
- *Make it harder:* Raise your top leg or arm.

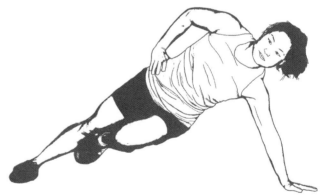

Side Plank & Knee Tuck

- Assume a Side Plank position on the floor.
- Tuck your bottom leg toward your chest.
- Hold the Plank with your leg raised for as long as you can.

Dynamic Side Plank

- Lie on your side on the floor with your upper body supported on one hand.
- Push through your hand and drive your pelvis to the ceiling.
- Stay active through your bottom leg as you raise your body up and down.

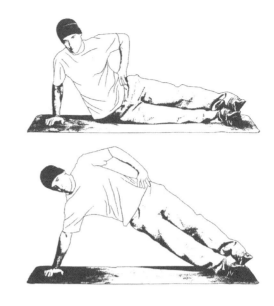

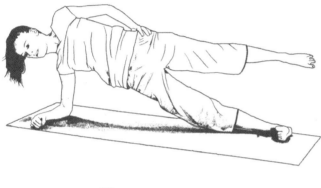

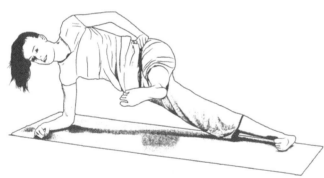

Side Plank & Leg Swing

- Place one forearm on the ground and get into a Side Plank position.
- Stay tight through your core and bottom leg, and then begin swinging your top leg forward and backward.
- Don't let your body rotate or fall over due to the leg motion.

Supine Plank

- Sit on the ground with your hands by your hips and your legs extended in front of you.
- Drive your hips to the ceiling to straighten your body into a single line from your shoulders to ankles.

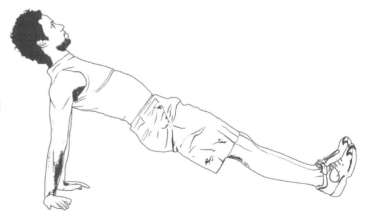

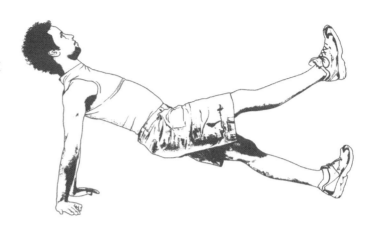

3-point Supine Plank

• Get on the ground in the Supine Plank position just described.

• Raise one leg off the floor as high as you can.

• Stay tight through your shoulders, core, and hips.

• Maintain the position for as long as possible.

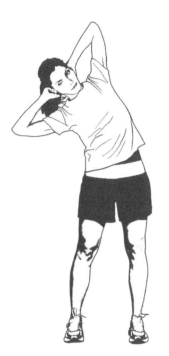 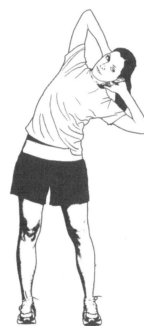

Standing Side Bends

• Stand with your feet shoulder-width apart and place your hands on the back of your head.

• Tighten your abdominal muscles and drop one shoulder to the side.

• Alternate side-bends between left and right without letting your trunk rotate.

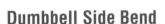

Dumbbell Side Bend

• Stand with your feet shoulder-width apart and hold a single dumbbell on one side of your body.

• Tip your body to the side holding the dumbbell, and then pull back up to the middle.

• Switch the dumbbell to the opposite hand and repeat on the other side.

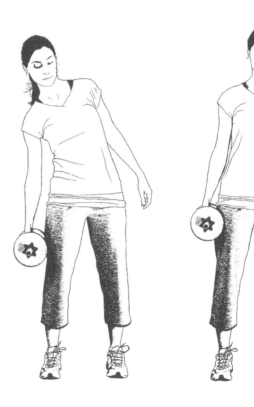

Saxon Side Bend

- Hold a weight plate above your head with your arms extended.
- Tip the weight to one side, allowing your trunk to perform a side bend.
- Tighten your abdominal muscles to pull yourself back up to midline.
- Repeat on the opposite side.
- *Variation:* Hold a dumbbell or medicine ball as resistance.

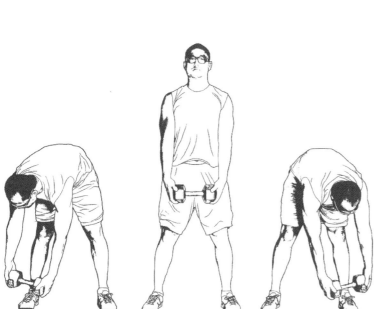

Alternating Toe Touch

- Stand with your feet slightly wider than shoulder-width apart while holding a dumbbell in front of your pelvis.
- Lower the dumbbell to one side, toward your foot.
- Engage your back muscles to lift your trunk back up to standing.
- Repeat on the other side.

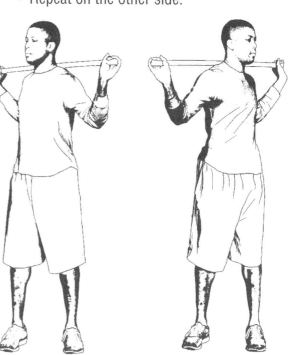

Trunk Twist with Bar

- Stand with your feet shoulder-width apart, holding a dowel or barbell behind your shoulders.
- Tighten your abdominal muscles and twist your trunk to one side.
- Return to the middle and then twist to the other side.

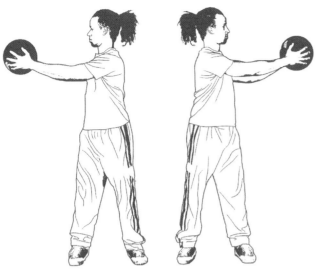

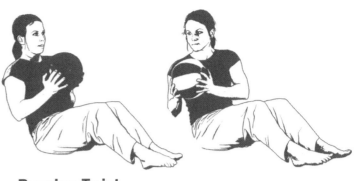

Med Ball Trunk Twist

- Hold a medicine ball at chest level, arms-length away from your body.
- Stay tight through your core and swing the ball from left to right.
- *Variation:* Keep the ball closer into your body.

Russian Twist

- Sit on the floor with your knees bent while holding a medicine ball at your chest.
- Tighten your core and begin twisting side to side with the ball.
- Keep your spine elongated while you twist.
- *Variation:* Hold a dumbbell or weight plate and try to keep your arms farther from your body.

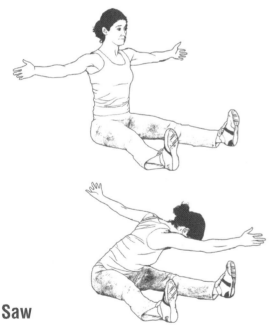

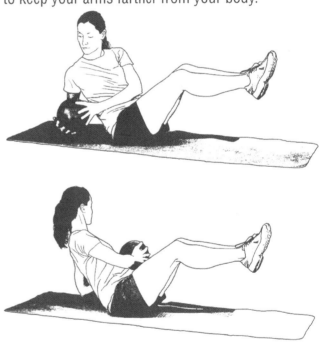

Saw

- Sit on the ground with your legs spread apart.
- Elongate your spine and reach your arms wide.
- Engage your abdominal muscles and bend forward, reaching one hand to the opposite foot.
- Return to the starting position and repeat on the other side.

Russian Twist - Feet Elevated

- Sit on the floor, balancing on your butt with your feet held in the air.
- Hold a medicine ball in front of your body and twist side to side.
- Stay tight through your core and don't let your chest drop.

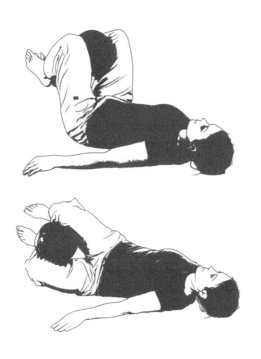

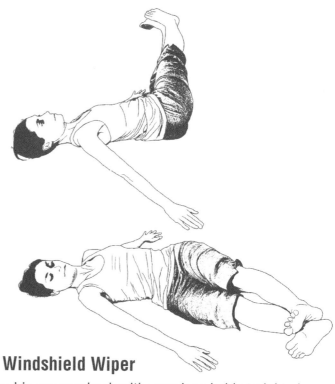

Floor Trunk Twist

- Lie on your back with your feet off the ground and your knees bent 90 degrees.
- Tighten your abdominal muscles and let your knees drop side to side in a twisting motion.
- *Make it harder:* Hold a medicine ball between your knees for extra resistance.

Windshield Wiper

- Lie on your back with your legs held straight above you.
- Tighten your abdominal muscles and let your legs drop off to one side, toward the floor.
- Reverse directions before your feet hit the ground, rotating back and forth like a windshield wiper.

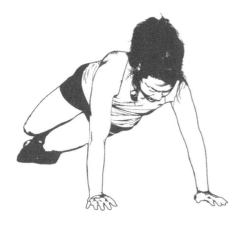

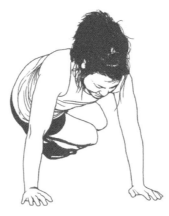

Quadruped Skiers

- Place both hands on the ground with your feet behind you and your knees doubled under you.
- Shift your weight into your arms and then hop your legs side to side, as if you were a mogul skier.
- Stay tight across your core as you rotate back and forth.

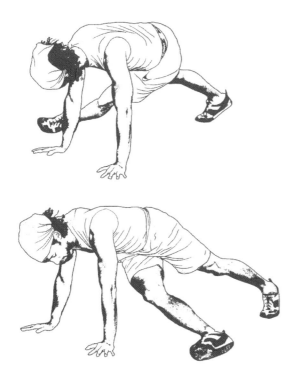

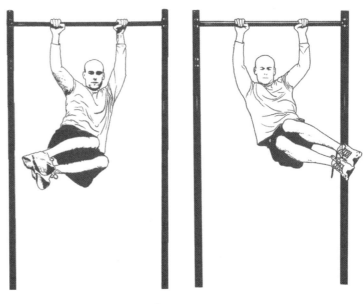

Hanging Trunk Twist

- Hang from a high bar with your knees pulled toward your chest.
- Tighten one side of your trunk and lift your legs to that side of your body.
- Lower your legs to the middle and repeat on the other side.

Quadruped Core Twist

- Place both hands on the ground with one leg extended backward and the other leg thrust underneath your lower body.
- Shift your weight into your arms and hop your legs from side to side, switching directions on each jump.

Hanging Windshield Wipers

- Hang from a high bar with your legs straight and lifted from your hips to 90 degrees.
- Allow your chest to drop backward to raise your legs higher.
- Rotate your pelvis from side to side so your legs move in a vertical plane, back and forth like windshield wipers.

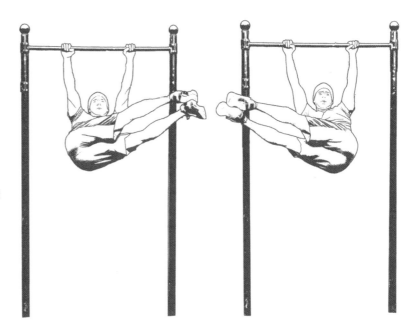

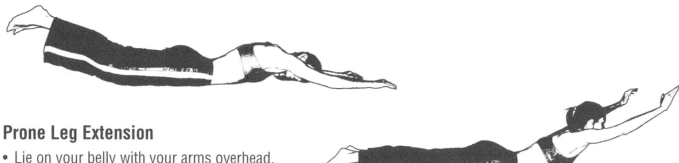

Prone Leg Extension

- Lie on your belly with your arms overhead.
- Tighten your hips and low back muscles and lift your legs off the ground.
- Raise your feet as high as you can, and then lower them back to the floor.

Prone Trunk Extension

- Lie on your belly with your arms raised overhead.
- Tighten your hips and low back muscles and lift your trunk off the floor.
- Lift your arms and sternum as high as you can before returning to the ground.
- *Variation:* Add rotation to the movement by looking over one shoulder and raising that arm higher than the other.

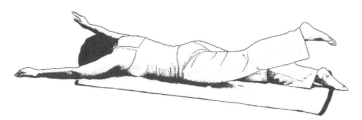

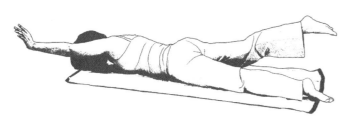

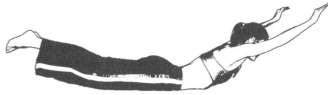

Prone Alternate Arm & Leg Lift

- Lie on your belly with your arms raised overhead.
- Tighten your hips and low back muscles, and then raise your opposite arm and your opposite foot.
- Raise them as high as you can before lowering them and repeating with the opposite limbs.

Prone Full Body Extension

- Lie on your belly with your arms raised overhead.
- Tighten your hips and low back muscles, and then raise your arm and your opposite foot.
- Raise them as high as you can before lowering them and repeating with the opposite limbs.

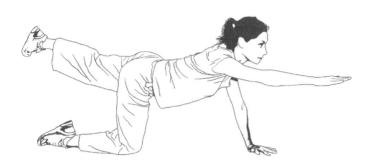

Alternate Arm & Leg Lift

- Kneel on the ground on all fours with equal weight between your hands and knees.
- Tighten your core and try to maintain a neutral spine position as you raise your arm and your opposite leg.
- Lift them as high as you can before lowering them to the ground and repeating with the opposite limbs.

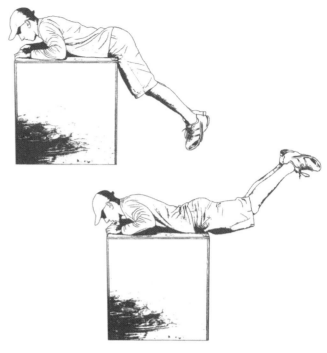

Reverse Hyperextension

- Position your chest and torso across the top of a plyo box, so your legs are hanging off one end.
- Tighten your hips and low back muscles, and then lift both legs up toward the ceiling.
- Raise your feet as high as you can before returning to the starting position.

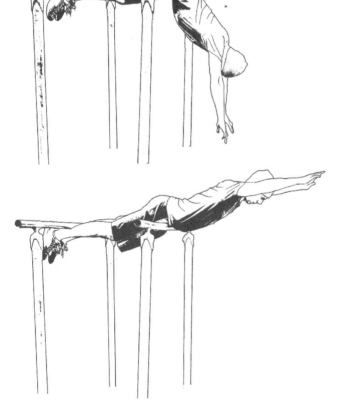

Hanging Back Extension

- Lie across a pair of parallel bars with your heels hooked under one bar and your pelvis supported on the other bar.
- Let your chest dangle downward to the ground.
- Tighten your hips and low back muscles, and then lift your torso upward to the sky.

Chapter 10

"It's time to explore some of the unique drills you can do with a stability ball."

Balls to the Wall

Big bouncy balls are the best. Don't laugh—I'm serious. You can actually do a ton of amazing strength and conditioning with a large, burst-proof plastic ball. Push your barbell and kettlebells to the side for a moment: It's time to explore some of the unique drills you can do with a stability ball (aka physioball or Swiss ball).

The first thing you need to know is that when you purchase a stability ball, you need to make sure to get the right size. Read the side of the box. It will tell you which size to get for your height and weight. Get too small of a ball and you'll be squirming around too much. Get too big of one and it'll be hard to position your body for optimal balance.

Now, for the real question I know you're asking yourself: Why do you need one of those big monstrosities in your home gym?

The answer couldn't be any more obvious: Stability!

You can take any of the upper body exercises—as well as a few lower body movements—and the planks seen in the previous chapters and perform them while positioned on top of a stability ball. The unstable platform of the stability ball forces you to engage your core muscles and other joint stabilizers more than if you performed the same movement on a firm surface.

Engaging a stability ball, rather than the floor or a classic weight bench, will challenge your body toward optimal performance because a higher degree of concentration is required to perform a given movement. You'll never have a personal record for bench or shoulder press on a stability ball, but it is one way to further prepare for the chaotic, unstable movements encountered during sports.

A few other key features of using a stability ball include the following:

- **Balance:** Just sitting on top of a stability ball requires extra effort to keep from falling over. By adding a balance challenge to a regular exercise movement, you increase its level of difficulty tenfold.

- **Core Strength:** Try to do anything on a stability ball without engaging your midsection and you won't be successful with the desired movement. You are forced to tighten your abdominal muscles.

- **Focus:** Because these balls are light and not tethered to the ground, they have a tendency to roll away from you if you're not paying attention. They force you to be present in your body and aware of how it is moving in space.

On top of these reasons, I also need to say that playing around on a stability ball is just a lot of fun. Do a quick YouTube search for stability ball tricks and you'll see what I mean. Rather than illustrate every single variation that can be performed on a ball, you'll see that the following pages give you a sample of the possibilities. The opportunities are limitless and you should feel free to make up your own challenging movements!

Stability Ball Crunch

- Support your trunk on a stability ball, with your feet flat on the floor.
- Tighten your abdominal muscles and lift your shoulders off the ball a few inches.
- Keep your hands either behind your head or across your chest.

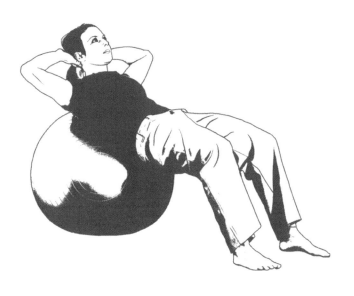

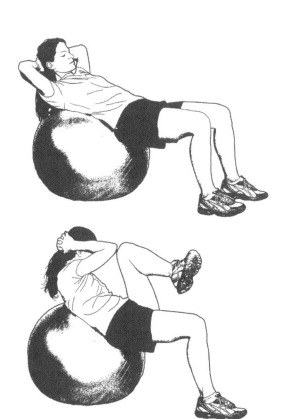

Stability Ball Elbow to Knee Crunch

- Support your trunk on a stability ball, with your feet flat on the floor.
- Tighten your abdominal muscles and lift your shoulders, bringing one elbow to your opposite knee.
- Alternate sides on each repetition.

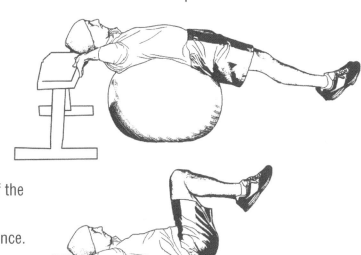

Stability Ball Reverse Crunch

- Lie on your back on a stability ball with your feet off the ground.
- Hold a weight bench or other firm structure for balance.
- Tighten your abdominal muscles and pull your knees into your chest.
- Stay tight in your core as you lower your legs back to a horizontal position.

Stability Ball Oblique Crunch

- Position your body sideways on a stability ball, with your feet tucked against a wall for support.
- Engage your core and hip muscles to lift your trunk off the ball.
- Elevate your chest as high as you can before lowering back to the ball.

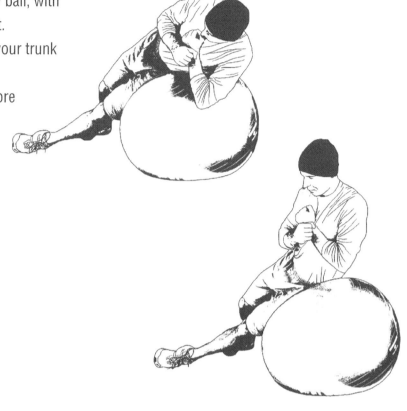

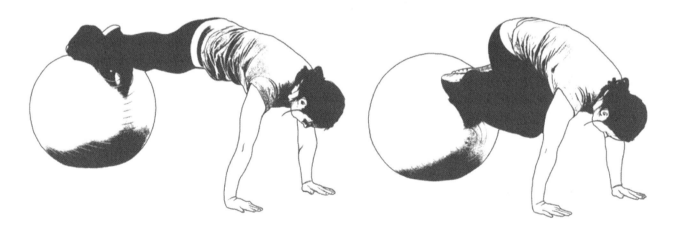

Stability Ball Jackknife

- Place your feet on a stability ball, with your trunk extended and hands flat on the floor.
- Shift your weight forward onto your shoulders and pull your knees into your chest.
- Stay horizontal as you push your legs back to the starting position.

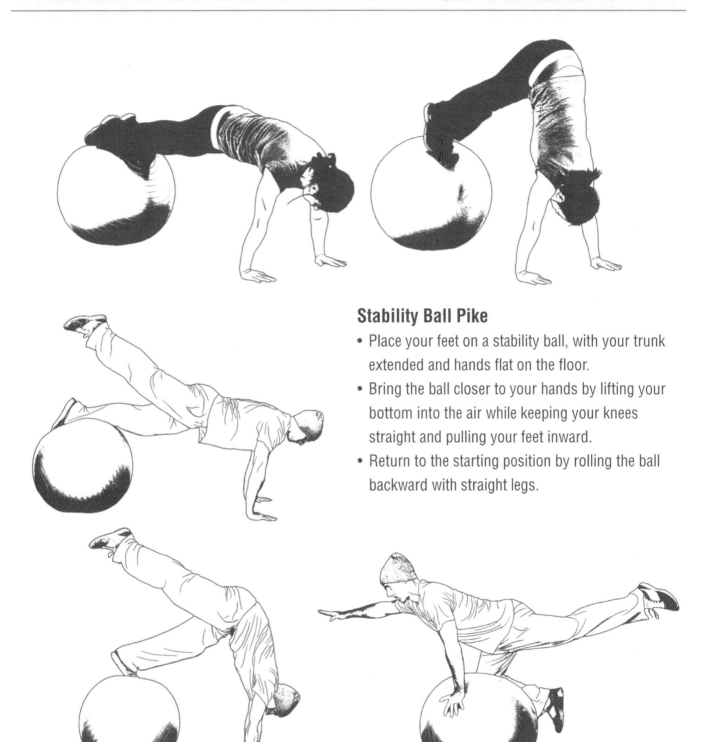

Stability Ball Pike

- Place your feet on a stability ball, with your trunk extended and hands flat on the floor.
- Bring the ball closer to your hands by lifting your bottom into the air while keeping your knees straight and pulling your feet inward.
- Return to the starting position by rolling the ball backward with straight legs.

Stability Ball Single Leg Pike

- Perform the same Stability Ball Pike just described, but keep one leg off the ball, elevated in the air.
- Avoid rotation in your trunk and lower body by staying extra tight through your shoulders and core.

Stability Ball Bird Dog

- Balance on your hands and knees on a stability ball.
- Try to lift one hand and the opposite foot.
- Hold for a few seconds, and then repeat on the other side.

Stability Ball Kneeling Twist

- Kneel on a stability ball, with your chest lifted as high as possible.
- Extend your arms away from your body, holding your hands together.
- Swing your arms from side to side while you stay balanced on the ball.

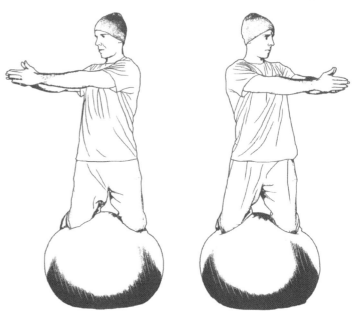

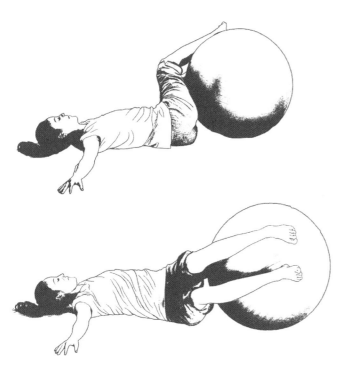

Stability Ball Hip Roll

- Lie on your back with your calves supported on top of a stability ball.
- Drop your knees from one side and then the other.
- Engage your core muscles to initiate the lower trunk rotation.

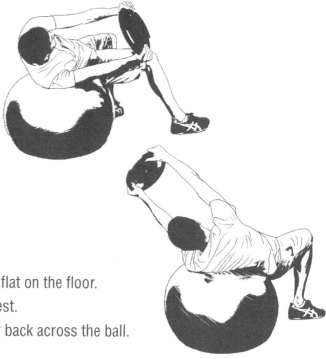

Stability Ball Weight Roll

- Place your upper back on a stability ball, with your feet flat on the floor.
- Extend your arms to hold a weight plate above your chest.
- Drop the weight from side to side, carefully rolling your back across the ball.

Stability Ball Skiers

- Place your shins on a stability ball, supporting your trunk with your hands flat on the floor.
- Tighten your abdominal muscles and rotate your lower body side to side.
- Keep your legs on the ball as you roll the ball back and forth.

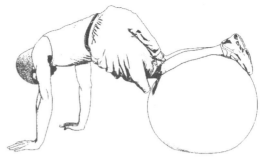

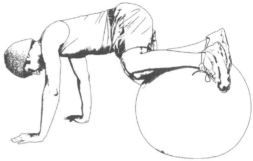

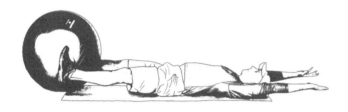

Stability Ball Pass

- Lie on you back, holding a stability ball between your feet.
- Lift your legs to bring the ball over your waist.
- Raise your trunk so that you can grasp the ball with your hands.
- Lower back to the floor, bringing the ball overhead.

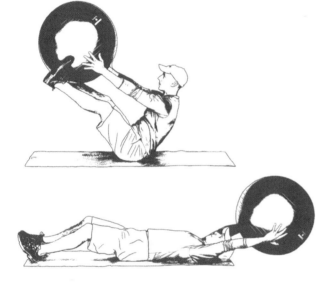

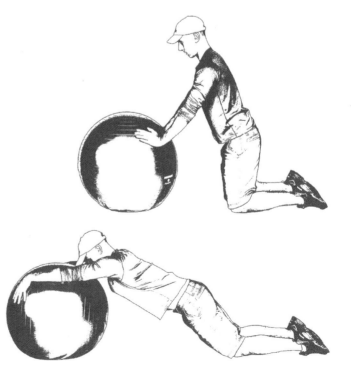

Stabilty Ball Roll-out

- Kneel on the ground with your hands placed on a stability ball.
- Tighten your core muscles and allow the ball to roll forward as you drop your chest to the floor.
- Reverse directions, lifting your trunk and pulling the ball back toward your hips.

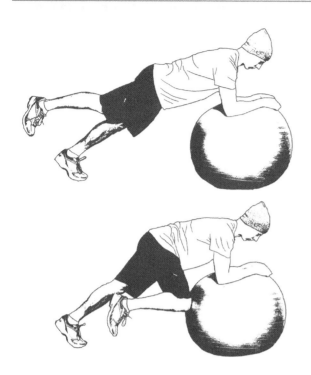

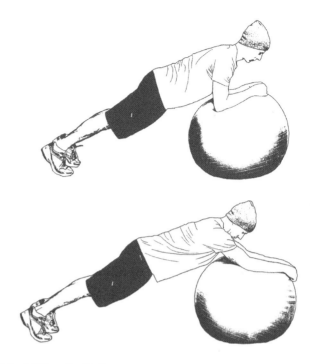

Stability Ball Plank Knee Drive

- Support your forearms on a stability ball, with your legs extended behind you in a Plank position.
- Lift one leg from the floor and drive that knee forward into the ball.
- Kick the leg backward into the air and repeat the "kneeing" motion.

Stability Ball Punch

- Support your forearms on a stability ball, with your legs extended behind you in a Plank position.
- Tighten your abdominal muscles and push your arms forward in a punching motion.
- Allow the ball to roll forward, and then reverse directions to bring it back under your chest.

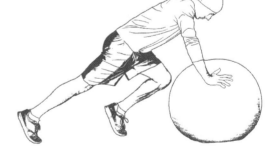

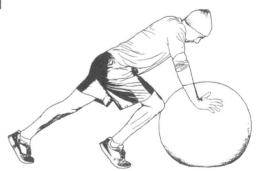

Stability Ball Mountain Climbers

- Place your hands on a stability ball, with your legs extended behind you in a Plank position.
- Alternate jumping your knees up to the ball, as if you were marching in place.
- Try to minimize as much motion in your upper body as possible.

Back Extension on Stability Ball

- Place your abdomen on a stability ball, with your feet tucked against a wall for support.
- Tighten your low back and buttocks to lift your chest from the ball.
- Lower chest over the ball again, allowing yourself to arch over its surface.

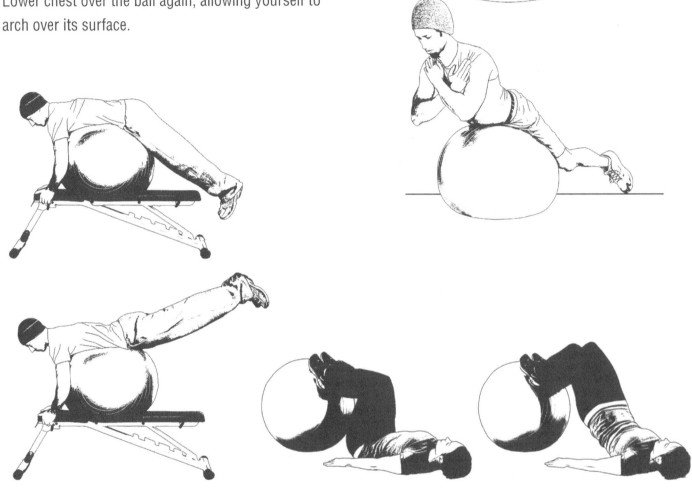

Stability Ball Reverse Back Extension

- Place your abdomen on a stability ball while holding onto a firm surface with your arms for support.
- Tighten your low back and buttocks to lift your feet from the ground.
- Raise your legs as high as you can before lowering them back to the floor.

Stability Ball Bridge

- Lie on the floor with your knees bent and your feet placed near the top of a stability ball.
- Tighten your core and push into your feet, lifting your waist from the ground.
- Elevate your pelvis as high as you can before returning to the floor.
- *Make it harder:* Try it with just one leg.

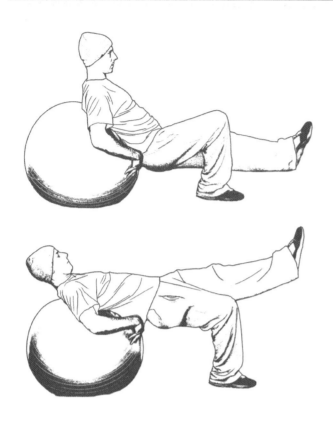

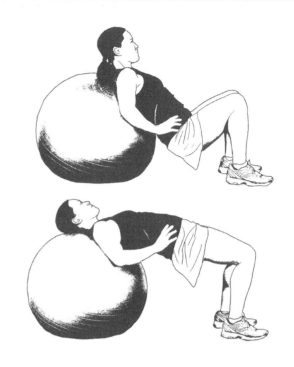

Stability Ball Single Leg Hip Thrust

- Support your upper back on a stability ball, with your hips bent and one foot on the floor.
- Hold one leg up in the air while you push the ground with your other foot.
- Lift your pelvis toward the ceiling.
- Go as high as you can before lowering back to the starting position.

Stability Ball Hip Thrust

- Support your upper back on a stability ball, with your hips bent and your feet placed flat on the floor.
- Tighten your hips and push your feet into the ground to lift your pelvis upward.

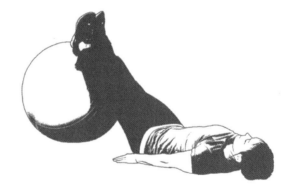

Stability Ball Pelvic Thrust

- Lie on your back with your legs straight and feet placed on top of a stability ball.
- Fire your core and hip muscles to lift your pelvis off the floor as high as you can.
- *Make it harder:* Hold one leg in the air.

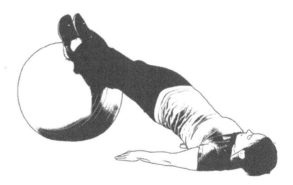

Stability Ball Wall Squat

- Rest your back against a ball that is placed against a wall.
- Bend your knees and roll the ball down the wall to achieve a deep squat.
- Fire your thigh muscles to press yourself back to standing.
- *Make it harder:* Try it with one leg or hold the bottom position for a longer time.

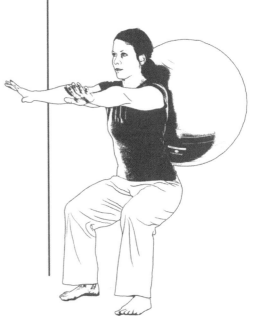

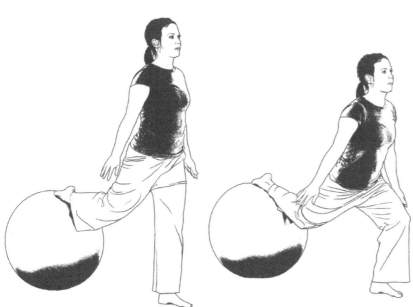

Stability Ball Split Squat

- Stand on one leg with your other foot behind you on the top of a stability ball.
- Stay balanced and lower into a single leg squat.
- Go as low as you can before rising back to the starting position.

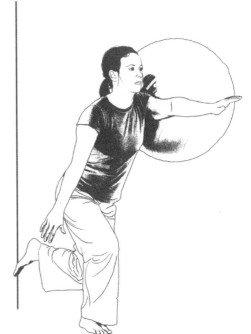

Stability Ball Lateral Wall Squat

- Place one shoulder against a stability ball positioned against a wall at chest height.
- Lift your inner leg from the floor and lower into a single leg squat while keeping pressure against the ball.
- Go as low as you can before pressing your outer leg into the floor to return to a standing position.

Stability Ball Leg Press

- Sit on the floor with your knees bent and back supported against a stability ball along a wall.
- Fire your legs to push backward into the ball so you rise to a standing position.
- *Make it harder:* Hold a weight plate or dumbbell for extra resistance.

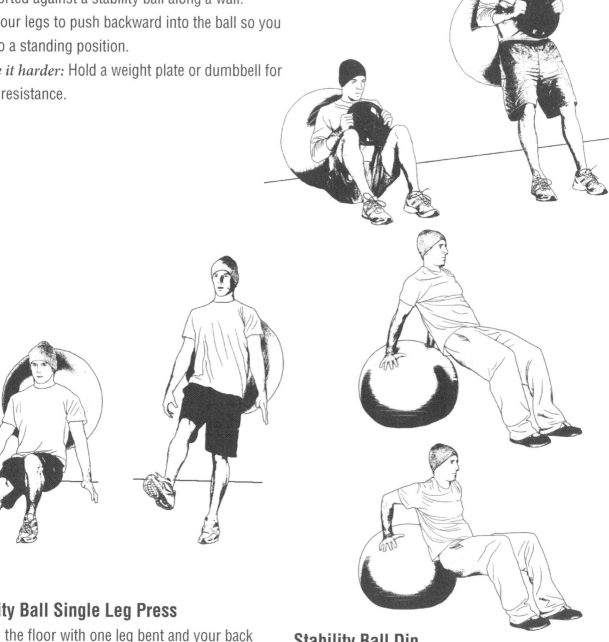

Stability Ball Single Leg Press

- Sit on the floor with one leg bent and your back pressing into a stability ball against a wall.
- Keep your other leg off the floor and push your bottom foot into the ground to lift yourself upward to the standing position.

Stability Ball Dip

- Place your hands on a stability ball behind you with your feet on the floor in front of you.
- Bend your elbows to lower your body downward.
- Press your hands into the ball to lift your chest back to the ceiling.

Bench Dip With Ball

- Balance with your hands on a bench behind you and your feet in front of you on a stability ball.
- Bend your elbows to drop your hips toward the floor.
- Press into your hands to raise your chest back up to the starting position.

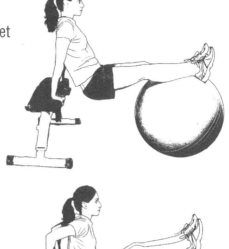

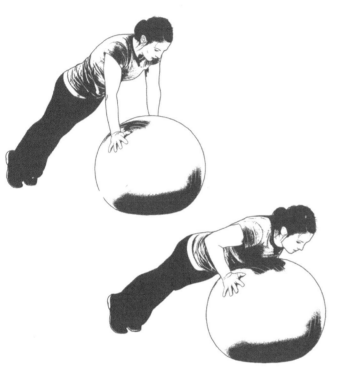

Stability Ball Push-up

- Place your hands on a stability ball, with your legs extended behind you in a Plank position.
- Bend your elbows and lower your sternum to the ball.
- Straighten your arms to push back up to the starting position.

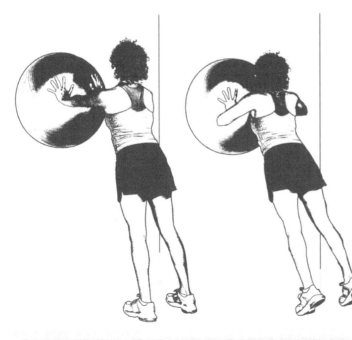

Stabilty Ball Wall Push-up

- Place your hands on a stability ball, positioned against a wall at chest height.
- Bend your elbows to lower your chest to the ball.
- Push into the ball to press yourself back to the starting position.

Stability Ball Decline Push-up

- Place your feet on a stability ball, with your trunk supported over your hands in a Plank position.
- Bend your arms to lower your chest to the floor.
- Straighten your arms to raise your trunk back to a horizontal position.

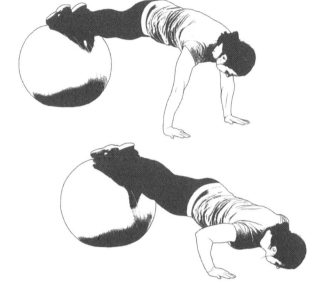

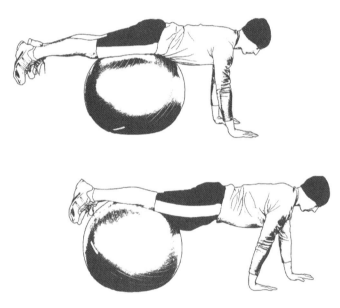

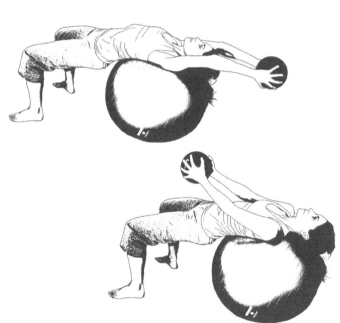

Stability Ball Walk-out

- Place your hands on the floor with your pelvis supported behind you on a stability ball.
- Stay tight through your trunk and walk your hands forward so the ball rolls down to your feet.
- Go as far as you can, then walk your hands backward, bringing your pelvis onto the ball again.
- *Make it harder:* Try walking your arms outward in a diagonal motion.

Stability Ball Pull-over

- Place your back on a stability ball, with your legs bent and feet flat on the floor.
- Hold a medicine ball over your pelvis and then lift it so it is completely overhead.
- Stay tight through your core as you lift the weight forward and backward.

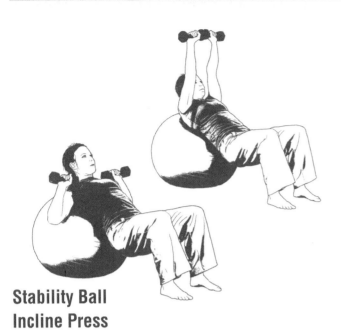

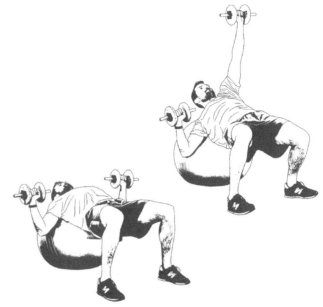

Stability Ball Incline Press

- Support your upper trunk on a stability ball, bending at your waist and keeping your feet flat on the floor.
- Hold two dumbbells at your shoulders and then press them to the ceiling.
- *Variation:* Sit on top of the ball to perform a true shoulder press.

Elbow Drive Press

- Support your back on a stability ball while holding two dumbbells near your shoulders.
- Drive one elbow into the ball while pressing the other hand to the ceiling.
- Allow your trunk to rotate as you push through your bottom elbow.
- Return to the starting position and repeat on the other side.

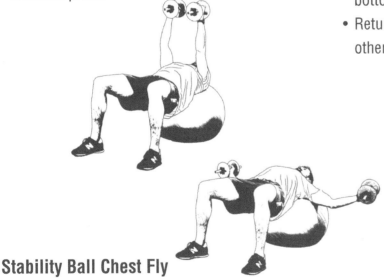

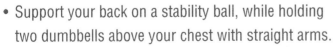

Stability Ball Chest Fly

- Support your back on a stability ball, while holding two dumbbells above your chest with straight arms.
- Spread your arms apart, lowering the dumbbells to the floor.
- Tighten your chest and core, bringing the weights back over your body.

Stability Ball Preacher Curl

- Rest your belly across a stability ball, with your elbows supported while holding a barbell in your hands.
- Lift the barbell to your face and then lower it back to the starting position.

Chapter 11

"There are a variety of exercises that simply cannot be done alone and teaming up with a partner is an awesome way to add spice to your workouts."

Team Up!

Two heads are better than one. Whether it's solving an engineering problem or working through a business transaction, having two people work on something always leads to a more complete solution. The same idea can be applied to your pursuit of fitness: Two bodies are better than one.

There are a variety of exercises that simply cannot be done alone and teaming up with a partner is an awesome way to add spice to your workouts. This chapter will give you nearly thirty partner skills to add to your movement repertoire.

Besides having a partner spot you on heavy lifts or challenging movements, there are plenty of ways that exercising with a companion can be beneficial. By combining your and your partner's body weight, you can add extra resistance to movements like squats and lunges. Likewise, a partner can either hold your legs to provide support or they can toss them to provide a challenging abdominal drill. Pitting your bodies against each other with push-ups immediately makes them harder, due to the extra instability. And, of course, how could you toss a medicine ball if it weren't for your workout buddy!

Exercising with a partner is plain fun.

Whether it's your best friend, a sibling, or a spouse, trying out new exercise movements together is bound to strengthen your relationship and bring a smile to your face. For safety's sake, keep good eye contact and communicate as much as possible so that no one gets hurt. When you begin to consider all of the cool moves you can do with a partner, you'll find that you never have an excuse to be bored at a party or while waiting for the bus!

Piggyback Carry

- Allow your partner to climb on your back, grasping her legs for support.
- Maintain this Piggyback position and carry your partner across the ground.
- Try to keep your chest elevated as you walk forward.

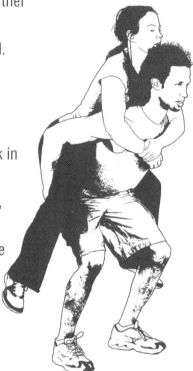

Piggyback Squat

- Allow your partner to climb on your back in a Piggyback position.
- Grasp her legs as you lower into a squat, and then return to the standing position.
- Don't lose the natural curve of your spine as you perform the movement.

Piggyback Side Lunge

- Let your partner climb on your back in a Piggyback position.
- Hold her legs for support as you step forward into a lunge.
- Push hard through your front leg to return back to the starting position.

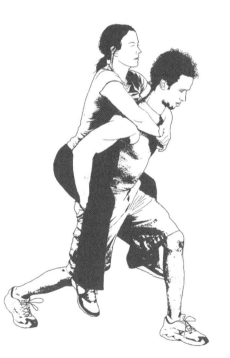

Piggyback Lunge

- Let your partner climb on your back in a Piggyback position.
- Hold his or her legs for support as you step forward into a lunge.
- Push hard through your front leg to return back to the starting position.

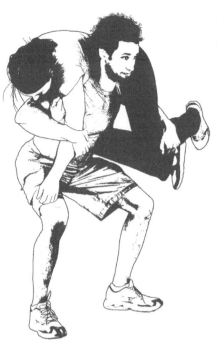

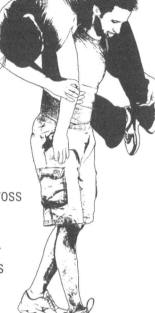

Fireman Squat

- Let your partner get on your back in a Fireman position, and hold her limbs for support.
- Maintain the curve of your lumbar spine as you lower your body into a squat.
- Return to standing.

Fireman Carry

- Have your partner drape herself across your upper back or shoulders, and hold her arms and legs for support.
- Keep her across your upper back as you walk across the floor.

Partner Air Squat

- Square off from your partner with your feet approximately 18 inches apart.
- Grasp one another's wrists and lower yourselves downward into a squat.
- Be careful to remain balanced, not pulling each other over too far, as you return to the starting position.

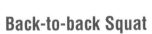

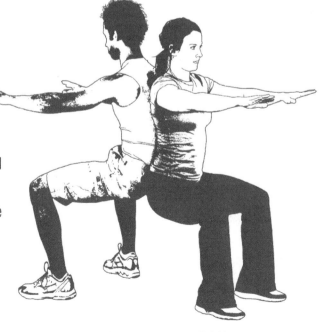

Back-to-back Squat

- Place your back in contact with your partner's back, and then walk your feet outward at least 12 inches.
- Press into each other as you lower your hips toward the floor, into a squat.
- Stay balanced as you push into one another and rise back to the starting position.

Glute Ham Tilt

- Kneel on the ground and have your partner press downward against your calves or ankles.
- Allow your body to sway forward a few inches before firing your glutes and hamstrings to return your trunk to vertical.
- *Make it harder:* Try to lower your body closer to the floor.

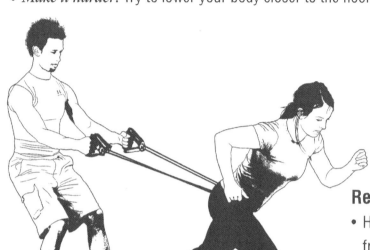

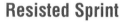

Resisted Sprint

- Have your partner hold a rope across your waist, from behind.
- Lean into the rope and begin to sprint forward as fast as you can.
- Your partner should keep pressure on the rope to try and arrest your motion.

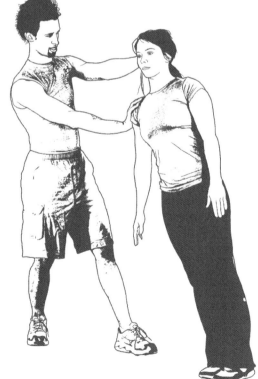

Partner Side Plank

- Lean sideways as your partner supports your upper body with his hands on your upper trunk.
- Stay balanced while holding the side plank for as long as you safely can.

Partner Get-up

- Lie on the ground with your knees bent and arms raised overhead.
- Your partner should sit over your feet and hold onto your calves.
- Swing your arms forward and lift your trunk into a sit-up.
- Have your partner pull forward on your calves to help you rise all the way to a standing position.

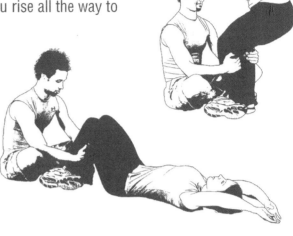

Leg Toss

- Lie on the ground and hold onto the ankles of your partner, who is standing above your head.
- Lift your legs to your partner, and then have him toss them to the ground.
- Stay tight in your abdomen and don't let your feet hit the floor.
- Lift your legs back to the starting position and repeat.
- *Variation:* Have your partner toss your legs off to the side.

Squat Toss

- Square off from your partner, at least a few feet apart.
- Lower into a partial squat and hold this position as you toss a medicine ball back and forth.
- Allow your trunk to rotate for an effective abdominal workout.

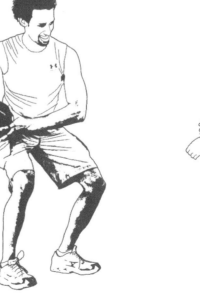

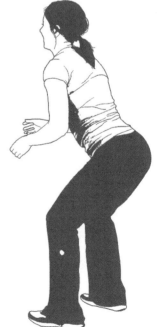

Lunge Toss

- Square off from your partner with at least a few feet between you.
- Hold a medicine ball at your chest, and then take a step forward into a lunge as you toss the ball to your partner.
- As your partner catches the ball, he should step backward into a reverse lunge before throwing it back to you.

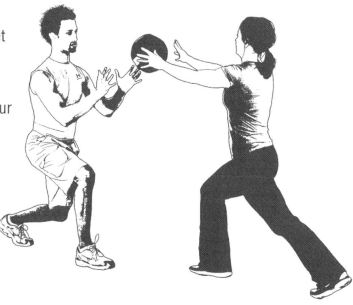

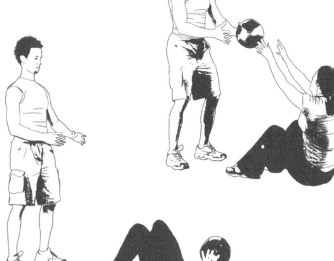

Sit-up Toss

- Lie on the ground with your knees bent and holding a medicine ball at your chest.
- Perform a Sit-up and toss the ball to your partner, who is standing a few feet away.
- When your partner tosses the ball back to you, catch it while sitting up, and then lower back to the floor to repeat the process.

Seated Toss

- Sit on the floor with your knees bent and with your partner standing at your feet.
- Toss a medicine ball back and forth between you while staying tight through your core and keeping your trunk off the floor.

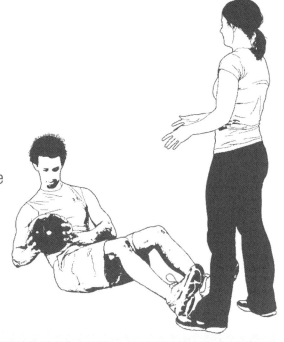

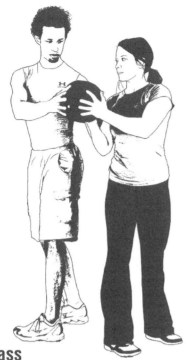

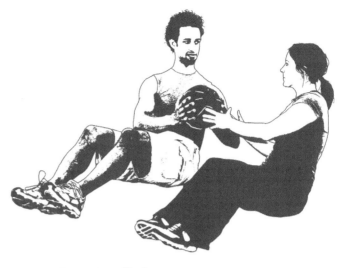

Partner Russian Twist

- Sit on the floor next to your partner, both of you bending your knees.
- Hold a medicine ball at your waist, and then turn your trunk and hand the ball to your partner.
- The partner will rotate to his opposite side and back to you.
- Take the ball and rotate to your opposite side, and then rotate back, returning the ball to your partner.
- *Make it harder:* Keep your feet off the ground.

Rotary Pass

- Stand back-to-back with your partner, holding a medicine ball at your chest.
- Turn to one side and hand the ball to your partner.
- Switch sides to have him pass it back to you.

Over Under Pass

- Stand back-to-back with your partner while holding a medicine ball.
- Raise the ball overhead and perform a slight back bend to pass the ball to her.
- Bend at your waist and reach between your legs as she passes the ball back to you.

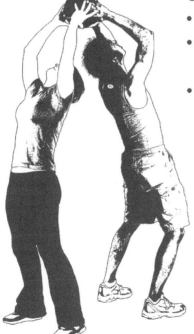

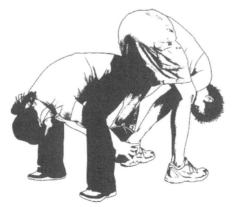

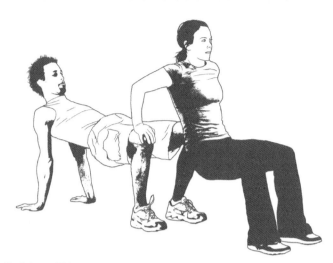

Bridge Dip

- Have your partner get on the floor, on all fours, with his chest toward the ceiling in a bridge position.
- Place your hands on his knees and perform body-weight dips.

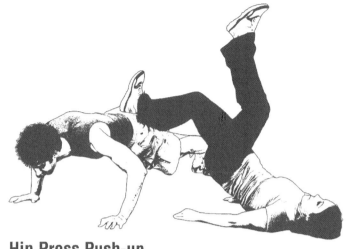

Hip Press Push-up

- Get into a Push-up position.
- Have your partner lie with her back on the floor and one foot on your sacrum.
- While you perform a push-up, your partner lifts her hips upward.

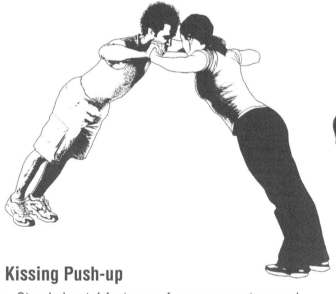

Kissing Push-up

- Stand about 4 feet away from your partner and grasp hands at shoulder height.
- Stay tight through your trunk and hips, and allow your elbows to bend in order to bring your head and chest closer together.
- Push into each other's palms to press back to the starting position.

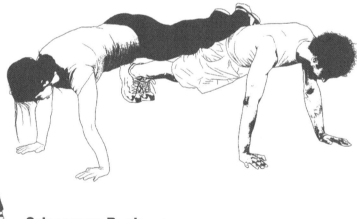

Crisscross Push-up

- Get on the floor in a Push-up position.
- Have your partner also get in a Push-up position, but turned 90 degrees and resting her feet on your low back or pelvis.
- Maintain this position while you lower and rise together, performing synchronous push-ups.

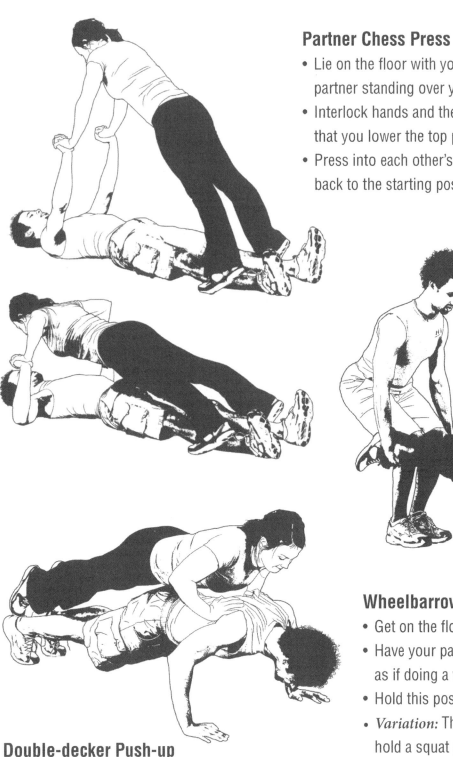

Partner Chess Press

- Lie on the floor with your arms extended and your partner standing over you.
- Interlock hands and then allow your elbows to bend so that you lower the top partner toward your chest.
- Press into each other's hands to push the top partner back to the starting position.

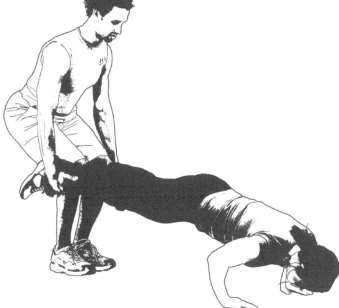

Wheelbarrow Push-up

- Get on the floor in a Push-up position.
- Have your partner grasp your ankles and lift them as if doing a wheelbarrow walk.
- Hold this position while you perform push-ups.
- *Variation:* The partner who is standing can try to hold a squat position.

Double-decker Push-up

- Get on the floor in a Push-up position and have your partner balance on your back, with her toes over your heels and her hands over your shoulders.
- Lower to the floor together and then press upward, while staying balanced.

Chapter 12

"Yoga practice is simply an excellent complement to all of the strength and conditioning you already do as an athlete."

Get Bent!

The practice of yoga postures has been around for well over one thousand years, and if you haven't taken at least one class, you, my friend, are out of the loop. Since the 1980s, yoga has snaked its way through Western culture to become a mainstream fitness activity, replete with studios in every neighborhood, dozens of practice styles, and a huge industry dedicated to keeping you outfitted in the right gear. But fear no yoga mat nor yoga pant: In this day and age, by practicing yoga you run no risk of being marked as a New Age fad follower. Yoga practice is simply an excellent complement to all of the strength and conditioning you already do as an athlete.

The benefits of yoga are numerous:

- **Flexibility:** Many postures demand that you contort your body into creative shapes, ultimately making you more limber.

- **Strength:** Yoga postures utilize your own body weight as resistance, but that doesn't mean they are easy. Holding your body off the ground rapidly becomes a challenge on par with many gymnastics-type strength feats.

- **Balance:** Whether you're balanced on one foot, your fingertips, or your rear-end, yoga postures force you to have command of your center of mass. A slight shift of your bulk and you can end up in a pile on the floor.

- **Core Support:** The instability present in many yoga postures demands that you be aware of the muscle action in your abdomen, hips, and low back. In a culture where back pain chases the common cold as the second or third leading cause for doctor visits, this is an excellent reason to take up yoga!

- **Physiological Effects:** The many inversions and twists unique to yoga can purportedly improve circulation and organ function, including digestion.

- **Relaxation:** It's widely accepted that exercise can help soothe the nerves, and yoga practice might just be the king of relaxation. Timing your breathing with slow-paced, methodical yoga postures is an excellent way to chill out.

The nuances of proper limb placement and alignment are extensive with yoga, and multiple pages could be written to describe the ideal performance of a given posture. Rather than getting derailed with identifying perfect form, this chapter is provided as a generic overview of 60 classic yoga postures. Go slow, don't expect miracles, and be gentle with your body (especially your neck). As a general rule, take your time to settle into the posture as best you can, and then try to hold the position for a set count of breaths.

Go and get bent!

Staff Pose

- Sit on the floor with your legs extended together in front of you.
- Elongate through your legs, from your heels to your sitting bones.
- Place your hands by your hips, tip your pelvis forward, and try to lift your spine vertically as high as you can.

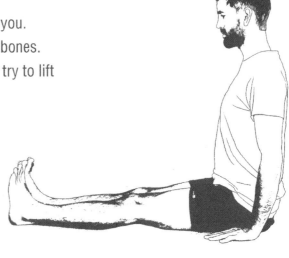

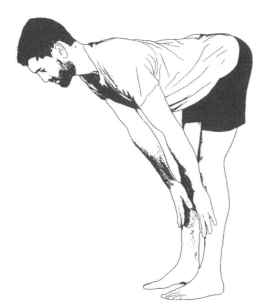

Standing Half Forward Bend

- Stand with your feet hip-width apart, tip your pelvis forward, and lower your chest into a forward bend.
- Maintain your back in a flat position and elongate through your legs, from your feet to your hip socket.
- Place your hands on your shins or thighs to assist the spine and leg position.

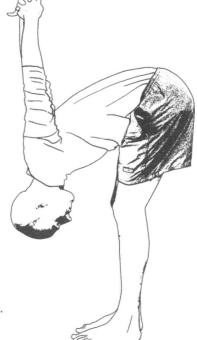

Clasped Arm Forward Bend

- Stand with your feet nearly touching and clasp your hands together behind your back.
- Bend forward and lift your arms to the ceiling, as high as you can go.

Downward-facing Dog

- Start with your feet about hip-width apart and your palms on the ground, a few feet in front of your toes.
- Tip your pelvis forward to maintain your lumbar curve while driving down through your heels and away through your fingers.
- Try to lengthen both halves of your body, lifting your hips into the air.

Scorpion Downward Dog Pose

- Perform the same Downward-facing Dog just described, but lift one leg off the ground.
- Pull the elevated leg higher and let it drop over the opposite side of your body.

Dolphin Pose

- Get in the same basic position as Downward-facing Dog, except place your forearms on the ground instead of your palms.
- Push through your arms while elongating through your legs to lift your pelvis into the air.
- Maintain your natural spine arch.

Child Pose

- Kneel on the floor and gently fold at your waist to bring your forehead to rest on the ground.
- Let your arms drape back to your feet and allow yourself to relax into this position.
- Drive your hips backward while softening your knees to compress your body even further.

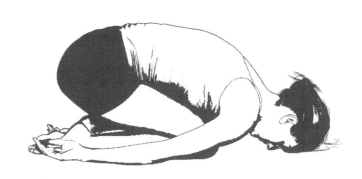

Extended Child Pose

- Get on the floor in the Child Pose as just described, but let your arms rest on the ground in front of you.
- Gently push through your arms while relaxing your knees and hips.

Pigeon Pose

- Position yourself on the ground with one leg extended behind you and the other leg folded in front of you, with the outer thigh and calf resting on the floor.
- Lower your chest to the ground without letting your front hip rise from the floor.

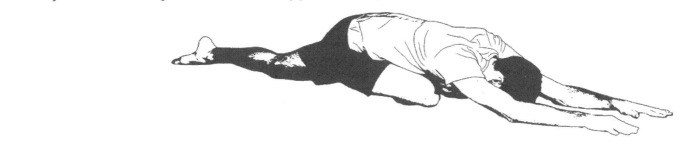

Extended Puppy Pose

- Kneel on the floor and place your arms on the ground in front of you.
- Drive your hips backward while elongating through your spine and reaching forward with your hands.

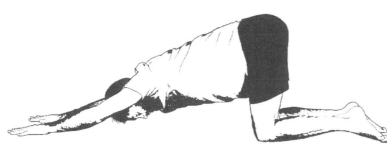

Reclined Cobbler Pose

- Lie on your back with your knees bent and the soles of your feet touching.
- Allow your hips to relax and let your knees spread apart.

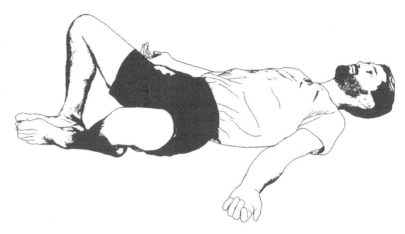

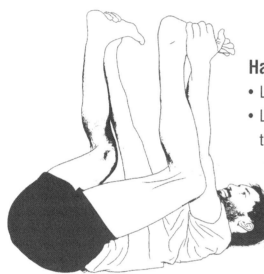

Happy Baby Pose

- Lie on your back, lift your legs, and grasp the outer edges of your feet.
- Let your hips open outward while providing some downward pressure through your hands into your feet.

Wide Legged Squat

- Squat on the ground with your hips spread wide and your feet rotated outward.
- Press your palms together and push your elbows into your knees so that your hips widen even more.
- Try to keep your back flat and elongated.

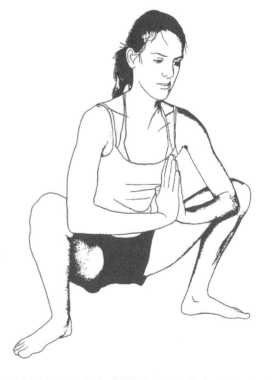

Frog Pose

- Position yourself on all fours on the ground, resting on your knees and forearms.
- Allow your legs to spread wide while gently pushing backward through your arms.

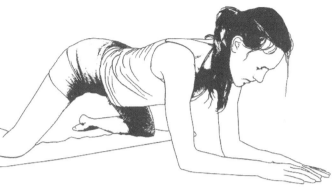

Wide Angle Seated Forward Bend

- Sit on the floor with your legs spread wide.
- Hinge forward from your waist while trying to keep your spine elongated.
- Grasp your feet to help pull yourself into a deeper bend and try to bring your belly flat on the ground.
- *Variation:* Try bending forward over just one leg at a time.

Intense Side Stretch

- Stand with your feet spread double shoulder-width apart.
- Rotate your hips so that both feet point to one side.
- Hinge forward and reach your hands toward the front foot.
- Drive downward through your back heel while keeping your spine straight and trying to bring your belly to your front leg.

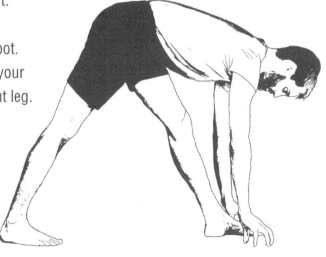

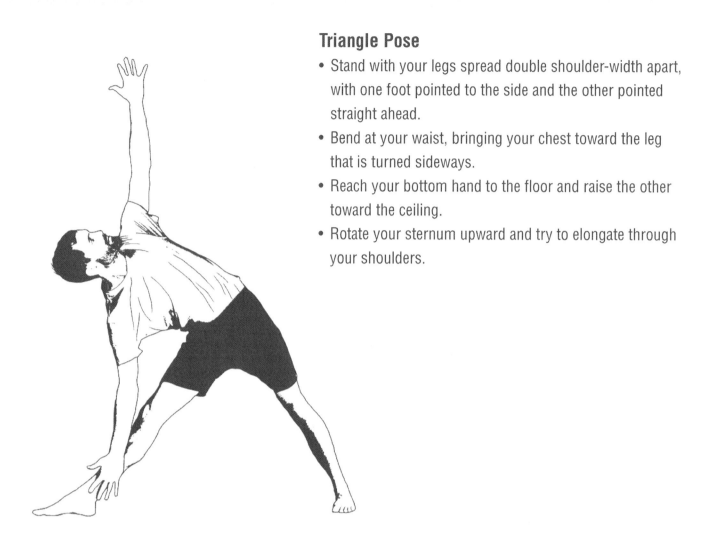

Triangle Pose

- Stand with your legs spread double shoulder-width apart, with one foot pointed to the side and the other pointed straight ahead.
- Bend at your waist, bringing your chest toward the leg that is turned sideways.
- Reach your bottom hand to the floor and raise the other toward the ceiling.
- Rotate your sternum upward and try to elongate through your shoulders.

Extended Side Angle

- Assume a low lunge, with the foot of the bent leg pointed to the side and the foot of the extended leg pointed forward.
- Drive the heel of your back leg to the floor.
- Hinge forward at your waist to bring your front hand near the outside of your front foot
- Reach your other hand overhead, lengthening from your fingertips to your back foot.

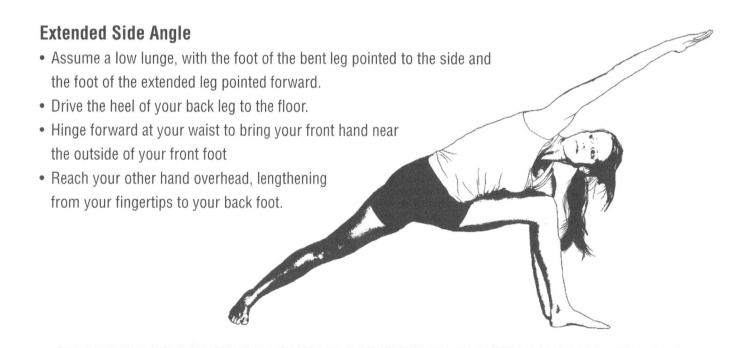

Bound Side Angle

- Start in the basic position of the Extended Side Angle.
- Drop your upper hand behind your back and reach between your legs to grasp it with your bottom hand.
- Rotate your chest to the ceiling and let your arms help pull you deeper.

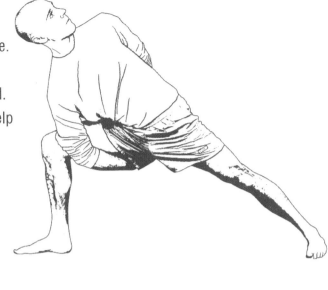

High Lunge

- Spread your feet apart in a wide lunge, with the heel of your back foot lifted off the ground.
- Raise your arms overhead, elongate your spine, and allow your pelvis to sink into the lunge.

Low Lunge

- Place the top of your back foot and shin on the ground and step your front leg forward into a deep lunge.
- Raise your arms overhead, lift your trunk, and allow your hips to sink into a deep stretch.

Warrior I Pose

- Step forward into a lunge, but drive your back heel into the floor with your toes pointed forward along a 45-degree angle.
- Keep your chest and pelvis rotated forward and lift your arms overhead.
- Elongate through your back leg and elevate your trunk as high as it will go.

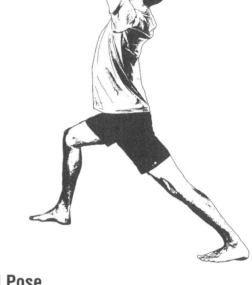

Warrior II Pose

- Start with the same foot placement as Warrior I, but let your pelvis and trunk rotate sideways.
- Extend your arms horizontally and try to flatten your body.
- Reach through your fingertips and drive strong through your feet.

Warrior III Pose

- Balance on one leg while extending your other leg backward and your arms overhead.
- Lower your torso to be parallel with the floor and extend from your fingertips to your toes.

Reverse Warrior Pose

- Place your feet on the ground in the same alignment as Warrior I.
- Reach your front hand up to the ceiling, tip your chest backward, and support your back hand on your rear leg.

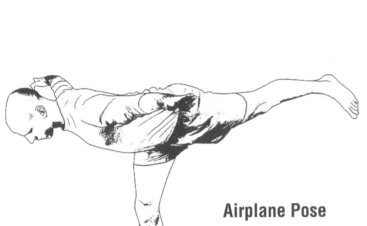

Airplane Pose

- Start in the same basic body position as Warrior III pose.
- Spread your arms wide like wings, rather than overhead.

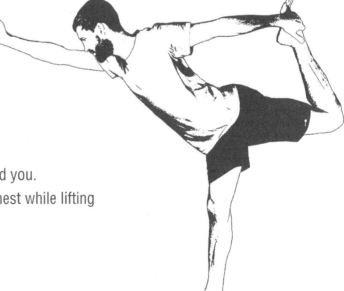

Dancer Pose

- Balance on one leg and grasp your other leg behind you.
- Extend your other arm overhead and lower your chest while lifting your back leg as far as it will go.

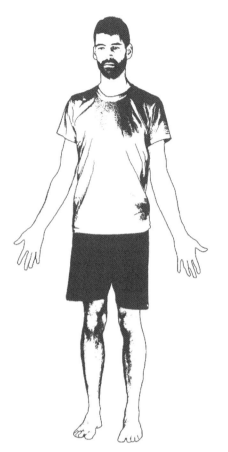

Mountain Pose

- Stand with your feet hip-width apart and your arms relaxed at your sides, palms facing forward.
- Be active through your feet and lift through your spine, elongating your torso as much as possible.

Tree Pose

- Balance on one foot while pressing your other foot into the inner thigh of your stance leg.
- Clasp your hands together, raise them overhead, and elongate from your toes to your fingertips.

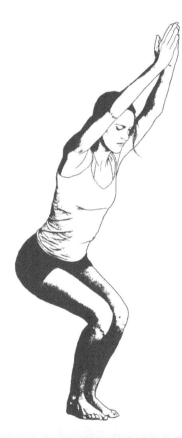

Chair Pose

- Stand with your feet and knees together while raising your arms together overhead.
- Lower your bottom into a semi-squat, as if you were sitting in a chair.
- Go as low as you can without losing the forward curve of your spine.

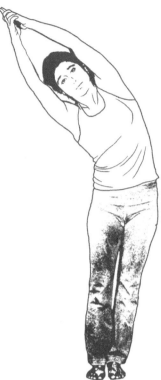

Half Moon Pose
- Stand with your feet together and hand interlocked overhead.
- Elongate your spine and bend to one side.

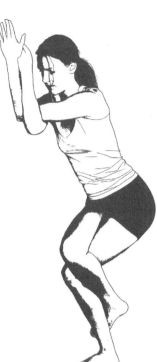

Eagle Pose
- Cross your elbows and interlock your forearms and palms.
- Balance on one foot and cross one thigh over the other.
- Lower down into a partial squat while keeping your arms and legs intertwined.

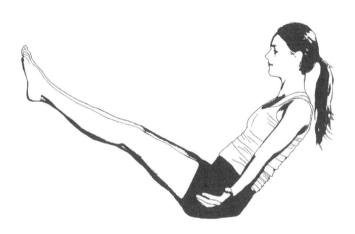

Full Boat Pose
- Sit on your bottom and raise both legs off of the floor to chest height, allowing your torso to drop backward 30 to 45 degrees.
- Stay tight in your hips and abdomen to balance in this position.
- *Make it harder:* Raise your arms overhead.

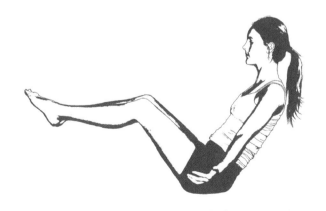

Half Boat Pose
- Sit on the ground in the same basic position as the Full Boat Pose.
- Allow your legs to bend so your feet are level with your knees.

Balancing Chalice

- Sit on the floor and grasp the arches of both of your feet.
- Hold your legs off the ground and extend them into wide splits.
- Keep tight in your abdomen and try to stay balanced in this position.

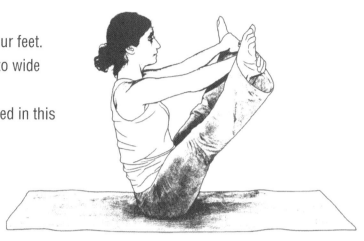

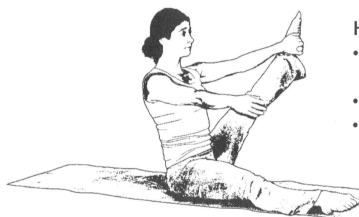

Half Chalice

- Sit on the floor with your legs straight and grasp the arch of one of your feet.
- Lift that leg off the ground and extend the knee fully.
- Keep your chest tall and try to stay balanced in this position.

Crane Pose

- Place your palms flat on the ground, shoulder-width apart.
- Raise your knees and place them on your elbows for support.
- Lift your feet from the ground, stay tight through your upper body, and balance on your hands.

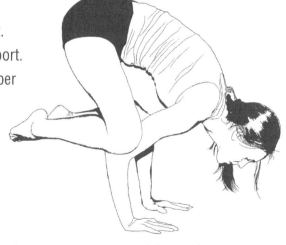

Seated Cross-legged Twist

• Sit with your legs crossed and spine elongated.

• Grasp one knee with your opposite hand and pull yourself into a twist.

• Inhale and elongate, exhale and rotate farther.

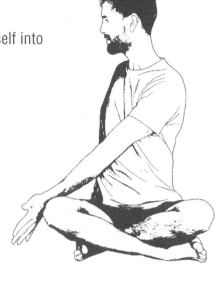

Revolved Standing Forward Bend

• Stand with your legs spread at least double shoulder-width apart.

• Reach one hand to the floor and rotate your trunk to the ceiling.

• Use your top hand to keep reaching upward, pulling yourself into a deeper twist.

Reclined Twist

• Lie on the floor with one leg straight and the other bent.

• Grasp your bent knee with your opposite hand and pull it over to the side.

• Keep your shoulders pressed into the ground and rotate your head toward your free hand.

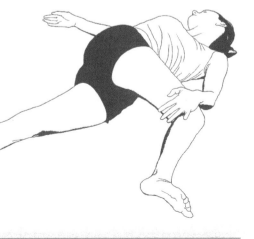

Revolved Forward Bend

- Sit on the floor with one leg straight and the other foot tucked into your inner thigh.
- Hinge forward at your waist to reach your front hand toward the toes of your extended leg.
- Use your free arm to reach up to the ceiling and rotate your trunk open to the side.

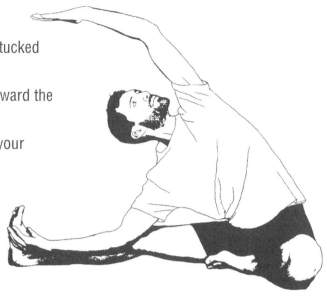

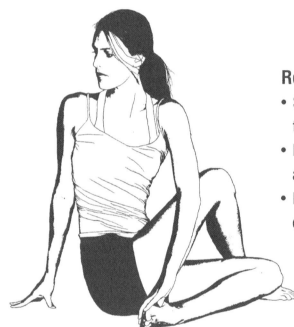

Revolved Seated Twist

- Sit with your legs crossed and the top leg elevated with the knee toward your chest.
- Reach the opposite arm across the elevated leg and apply gentle pressure to assist with moving into a twist.
- Inhale and extend your trunk, exhale and twist into a deeper rotation.

Bound Knee Twist

- Sit with one leg extended on the ground and the other flexed to your chest.
- Take the arm closest to the bent leg and wrap it around the knee and behind you.
- Rotate your torso to the opposite side.
- Reach behind your back with your free arm and try to grasp your hands.

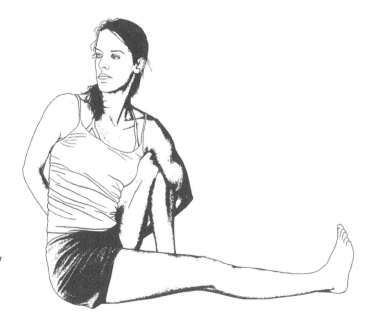

Mariachi's Pose

- Sit with one leg extended on the ground, cross the other leg over top, and bring your knee near your chest.
- Place your opposite elbow on the elevated knee and apply gentle pressure to help rotate your trunk to the side.

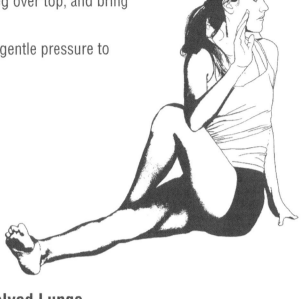

Revolved Lunge

- Step into a deep lunge, with the front knee bent and your back heel off the ground.
- Rotate your trunk to bring your opposite elbow to rest on the front knee, with your hands pressed together in a "prayer" position.
- Apply light pressure through your elbow to help rotate into a deeper twist.

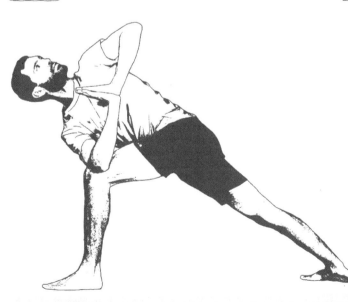

Revolved Side Angle

- Begin in the Extended Side Angle position, with your back heel on the ground and your foot angled forward 45 degrees.
- Press your hands together in a prayer position and rotate your trunk to bring your elbow to the outside of your front knee.
- Apply light pressure to help your chest rotate upward to the ceiling.

Revolved Chair

- Get in the Chair Pose previously described, with your palms pressed together in a prayer position.
- Place one elbow on your opposite knee and rotate your chest to that side.
- Press your elbow into your knee to take your trunk into a deeper rotation.

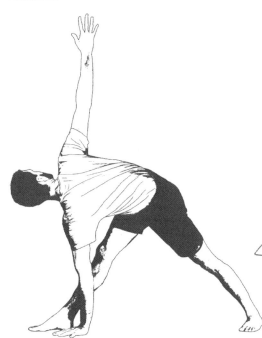

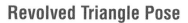

Revolved Triangle Pose

- Begin in Triangle pose, but rotate your trunk to bring your back hand to the instep of your front foot.
- Lift your front hand and rotate your chest to the ceiling.

Upward-facing Dog

- Lie on your belly with your hands placed at your sides, near your chest.
- Press your palms into the floor and lift your sternum upward.
- Raise your chest as high as you can, while pressing through your feet and allowing your pelvis to rise from the ground.

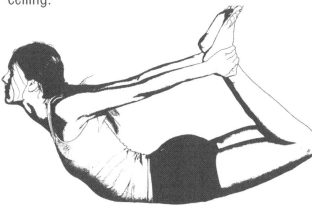

Bow Pose

- Lie on your belly, bend your knees, and reach your hands backward to grasp your feet.
- Lift your chest while simultaneously pressing your feet to the ceiling.

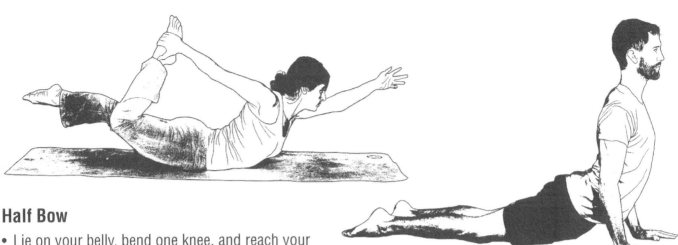

Half Bow

- Lie on your belly, bend one knee, and reach your hand back to grasp your foot.
- Lift your chest and press your hand and foot to the ceiling.
- Extend your other arm and leg, reaching out from your fingers and toes.

Cobra Pose

- Lie on your belly with your palms flat on the ground, positioned next to your ribcage.
- Push your hands into the floor and lift your chest, but keep your pelvis adhered to the ground.

Upward Plank Pose

- Sit on the floor with your legs extended and your hands flat on the ground behind your back and with your fingertips pointed behind you.
- Push into your hands and feet, drive your hips to the ceiling, arch your back, and drop your head backward.

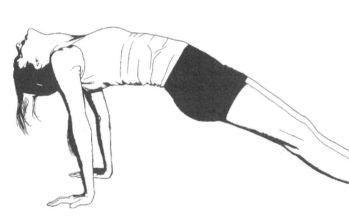

Bridge Pose

- Lie on the ground with your knees bent and your feet flat on the floor.
- Interlace your hands beneath your bottom.
- Push your feet into the ground and drive your hips to the ceiling.
- Your weight should be distributed between your shoulders and feet.

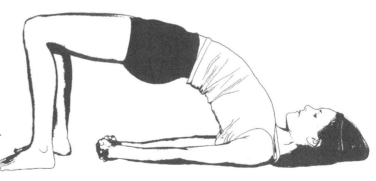

Extended Bridge

- Get in position to perform a Bridge Pose, but lift one leg from the floor.
- Drive your hips to the ceiling and lift your free leg to vertical while reaching through your toes.

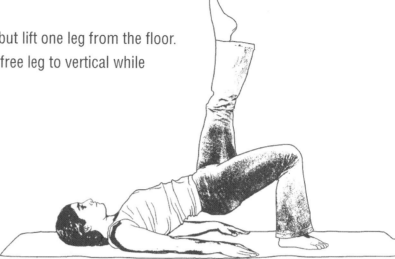

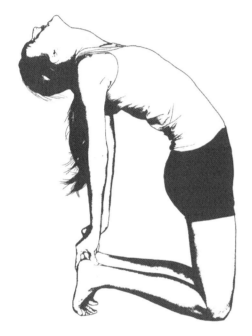

Camel Pose

- Kneel on the ground with your hips positioned over your knees.
- Reach your hands backward to grasp your heels, and push your hips forward.
- Let your back and neck extend into an arch while lifting your chest to the ceiling.

Wheel

- Lie on your back with your knees bent, feet flat on the floor, and your palms pressed into the ground next to your shoulders.
- Press into your hands and feet, lifting your pelvis and torso to the ceiling.
- Drive upward through your hips and shoulders, arching your back into a deep bend.

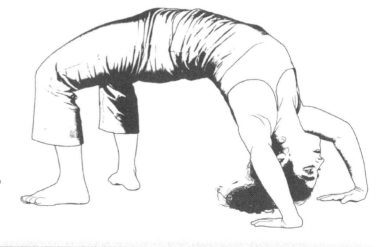

Fish Pose

- Lie on your back with your elbows on the ground, pressed against your ribs.
- Push down into your elbows while lifting your chest upward and dropping your head toward the floor.

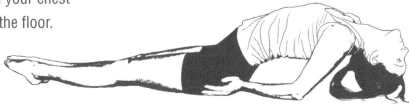

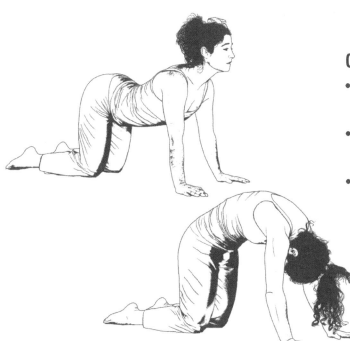

Cat Cow

- Kneel on all fours with your weight evenly distributed between your hands and knees.
- First, let your belly sag toward the floor completely and lift your head to the sky.
- Second, drop your head and reverse the arch of your spine, lifting your back upward to the ceiling as high as you can.

Locust Pose

- Lie on your belly with your arms extended at your sides, by your hips.
- Tighten your back and hips to lift both your chest and feet from the ground as high as you can.

Half Locust Pose

- Lie on your belly with your arms extended and palms pressed into the floor by your hips.
- Tighten your back and hip muscles to lift your feet from the floor as high as you can.

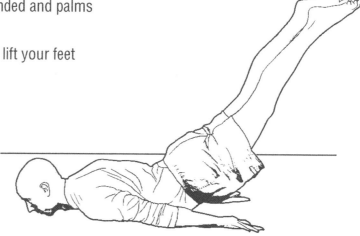

Rabbit Pose

- Kneel on the floor and bend forward to carefully place the top of your head on the floor.
- Lift your hands and arch your back, raising your spine to the ceiling.

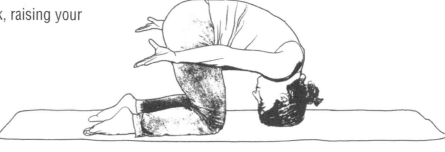

Plow Pose

- Lie on your back with your arms extended by your sides.
- Gently raise your legs and pelvis, taking them completely overhead to reach your toes to the ground behind you.

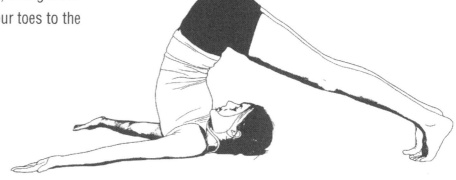

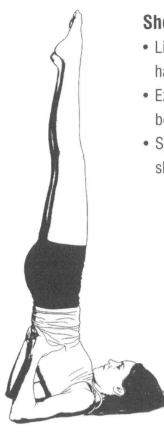

Shoulder Stand

- Lie on your back with your hips raised and your hands placed on your low back for support.
- Extend your feet to the ceiling to make your lower body into a vertical line.
- Spread your weight evenly between your elbows and shoulders, with no pressure on your neck.

Forearm Stand

- Place your forearms on the floor with your body in a pike position beneath you.
- Carefully lift your legs directly overhead while balancing on your forearms, and with no pressure on your head.

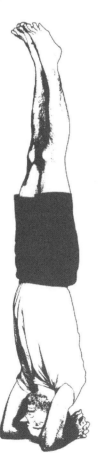

Head Stand

- Place your head on the ground with your forearms on either side of it, in a tripod position with three points of your body on the floor.
- Lift your legs directly overhead while balancing in the tripod position.
- Reach your toes to the ceiling to elongate your body.

Chapter 13

"When used correctly, stretching is fundamental upkeep for the athletic body."

Unwind

t's funny how times change. If *Mad Skills* had been written in the 1980s, this chapter probably would have come at the beginning of the book. Alas, it's 2013 and we now have a bit more insight into the role of stretching on human performance. Static stretching before being active or working out has lost favor, due to ineffectiveness and the potential for actually impairing performance. The concept hasn't yet been forgotten in the dustbin of history, but the role of stretching in fitness and athletics has certainly changed.

Stretching is the purposeful elongation of muscle tissues with the hope of achieving a sustained change in tissue length. It's done to loosen tight structures, but it's not the end-all-be-all of improved joint function. Witness the rise in popularity of the term "mobility", and the use of foam rolls, lacrosse balls, and bands to help restructure tissues and promote better movement.

So, what is the role of stretching for today's athlete and fitness enthusiast? Why even include it in this exercise encyclopedia?

When used correctly, stretching is fundamental upkeep for the athletic body. Repetitive movement, heavy weight lifting, and extreme physical challenge inevitably cause muscles to tighten in predicable patterns. Without appropriate focus, this muscle tightening will lead to restricted motion and postural changes. Translation: Game over for performing at your highest capacity.

A strong and stiff body is no better off than a weak and flexible body. You need both: flexibility and strength.

Stretching is still and will likely always be one key way for you to keep your body supple and prepared for the unique physical challenges. Aside from helping you maintain normal posture and joint motion, it will also help you prevent injury. Changes in posture and muscle length place your body at risk for a variety of painful injuries such as a strain or tendonitis. Routine stretching can help prevent them.

Assuming you're convinced, let's move on with two essential rules:

1. **Never stretch a cold muscle.** Think of your muscles like Silly Putty. You can only elongate them when they are thoroughly warmed up. Either stretch after your workout or athletic event or do 10 minutes of a general warm-up prior to exercising. (Refer to Chapter 1 for warm-up ideas.)

2. **Hold each stretch for sufficient duration.** For tissue elongation to happen, you need to spend a sustained amount of time in the stretch. At a minimum, shoot for 15 seconds in a position. If possible, strive for 30 to 60 seconds. If you just move in and out of a stretch rapidly, you are doing nothing of benefit for your body.

A third item that is worth considering is that you shouldn't be afraid of including a few dynamic elements in your stretching routine. For example, having a parter push or pull you into a deeper stretch can be a nice way to gain extra flexibility. Holding a weight can be another way you can help yourself lower into a few positions. Similarly, by contracting and then relaxing the opposing muscle group for a given stretch, you can often sink farther into your available range of motion.

There are 70+ stretches illustrated in this chapter. Keeping in line with the M.O. of *Mad Skills,* the greater variety of movements you are competent with (stretches in this case), the better athlete you will be. Depending on your current fitness blueprint, some stretches might be essential, while others are less necessary. If your favorite sport is heavy in one muscle group, then spend extra time with the stretches for that body part. Cyclists are a great example—often needing extra attention to their quads, hamstrings, and hip flexors.

Clear out some space on the floor. Make room to relax. Unwind and restore your body's flexibility.

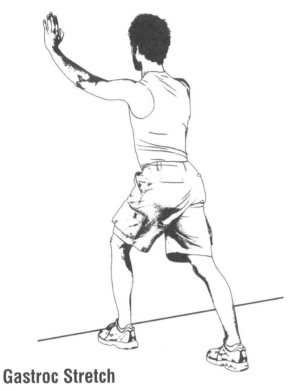

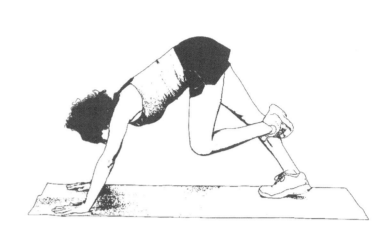

Gastroc Stretch

- Place one leg behind you with your knee straight and heel on the ground.
- Support your arms on a wall or railing.
- Drive your back heel downward while bringing your hips forward.

Bent Over Calf Stretch

- Place both hands on the ground, and put one foot behind you and lift the other from the floor.
- Press your heel downward to feel a stretch in your calf.

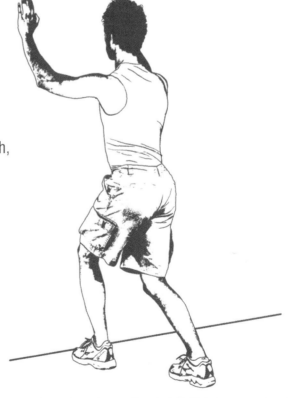

Soleus Stretch

- Perform the same basic movement as the Gastroc Stretch, but allow the knee of your back leg to bend.
- You should feel the stretch lower and deeper in your calf.

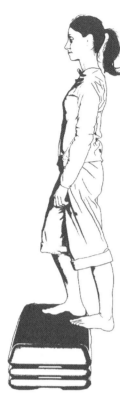

Stair Stretch

- Stand on the edge of a stair and allow one heel to hang over the edge.
- Keep your foot supported toward the toes.
- Drive your heel down to the floor to feel the stretch.

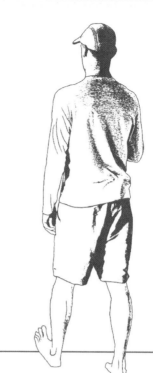

Wall Foot Stretch

- Place your toes and the ball of one foot up against a wall.
- Lean into the wall to feel the stretch in your arch and calf.

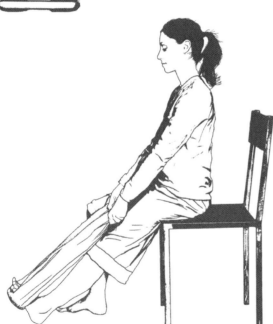

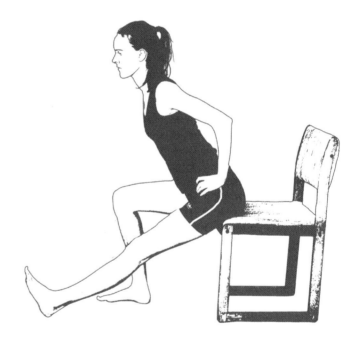

Towel Foot Stretch

- Sit near the edge of a chair and loop a towel or strap around the ball of one foot.
- Extend your leg and pull the towel upward, bringing your toes toward your face.

Seated Hamstring Stretch

- Sit at the edge of a chair, with one leg extended in front of you and your heel on the ground.
- Grasp the bones at the front of your waist and tip your pelvis forward.
- Don't let your spine lose its arch.

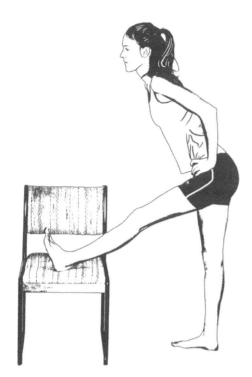

Standing Hamstring Stretch

• Stand and place one heel on chair, keeping your knee extended.

• Tip your pelvis forward to feel a stretch on the underside of your thigh.

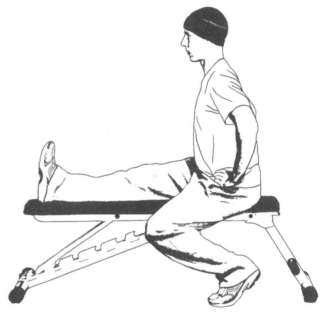

Supported Hamstring Stretch

• Sit with one leg extended along the top of a bench.

• Rest your other leg off to the side.

• Tip your pelvis forward to engage a stretch of your hamstrings.

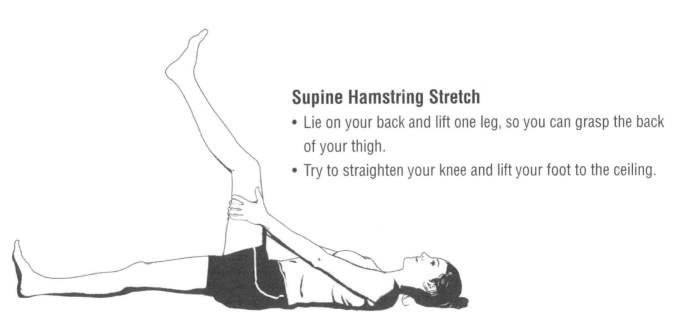

Supine Hamstring Stretch

• Lie on your back and lift one leg, so you can grasp the back of your thigh.

• Try to straighten your knee and lift your foot to the ceiling.

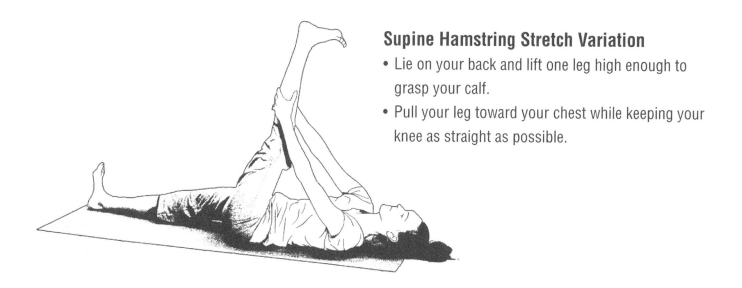

Supine Hamstring Stretch Variation

- Lie on your back and lift one leg high enough to grasp your calf.
- Pull your leg toward your chest while keeping your knee as straight as possible.

Hamstring Stretch with Strap

- Lie on your back and place a strap around the arch of one foot.
- Pull the strap to lift your leg to the ceiling while keeping your knee straight.

Wall Hamstring Stretch

- Lie on the ground, straddling a doorframe or the corner of a wall.
- Place one foot the wall and let your other leg run straight along the ground.
- Slide your foot up the wall while scooting your hips closer to the wall.

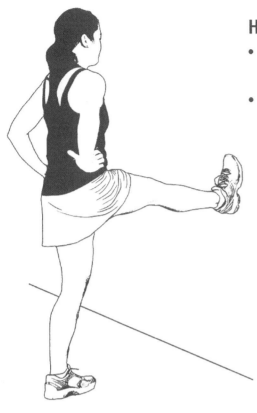

Hamstring Stretch at Wall

- Place one foot flat against a wall at close to hip-height, keeping your knee straight.
- Tip your pelvis forward to feel a stretch in your hamstrings.

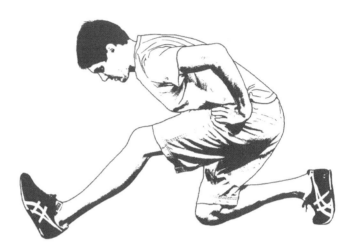

Kneeling Hamstring Stretch

- Kneel on one knee with your other leg extended in front of you.
- Try to straighten the knee of your front leg while tipping your pelvis forward.

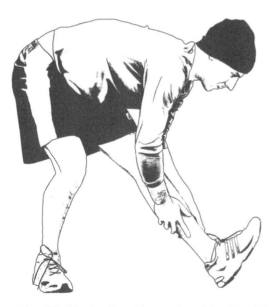

Squat Hamstring Stretch

- Stand with your legs almost double shoulder-width apart.
- Place the heel of one foot on the ground and rotate your body toward that leg.
- Straighten your knee while bending forward from your waist, bringing your chest toward the outstretched leg.

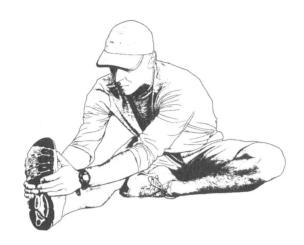

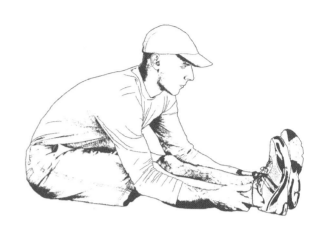

Single Leg Forward Bend

- Sit on the ground with one leg extended and the other leg bent with its foot tucked into your thigh.
- Tip your pelvis forward and reach for the toes of your outstretched leg.

Double Leg Forward Bend

- Sit on the ground with both legs outstretched in front of you.
- Hinge forward through your waist, reach for your toes, and try to bring your chest closer to your thighs.

Standing Quad Stretch

- Balance on one leg, grasp the top of your opposite foot, and pull your heel toward your bottom.
- Hold a wall for balance, as needed.
- Try to keep your knee pointed toward the ground.

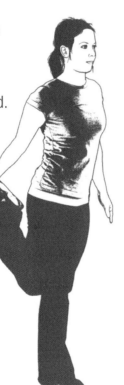

Supported Quad Stretch

- Place the top of one foot on a box or bench, keeping your knee flexed and pointed toward the ground.
- Gently ease your hips backward and downward to bring your bottom closer to your heel.

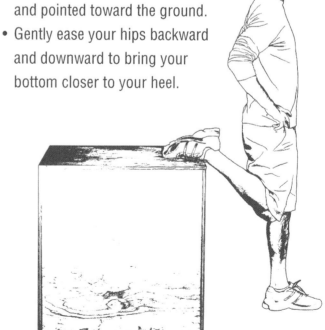

Side Lying Quad Stretch

- Lie on your side and bend your top leg.
- Grab the top of your foot and pull your heel toward your bottom.

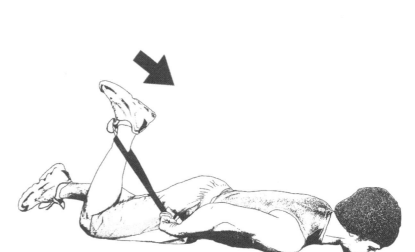

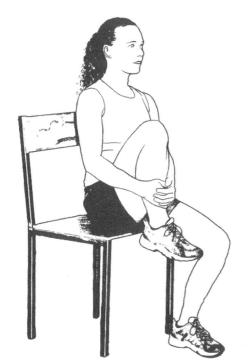

Knee Flexion Stretch - Sitting

- Sit at the edge of a chair and grasp the shin of one leg.
- Pull your heel toward your bottom, as far as it will go.

Prone Knee Flexion with Strap

- Lie on your belly with a strap placed around the ankle of one leg.
- Pull the strap to bring your heel closer toward your bottom.
- Don't let your pelvis rise off the floor.

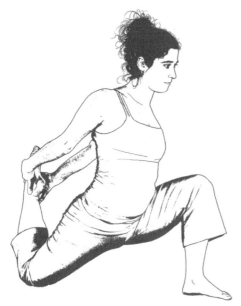

Deep Quad Stretch

- Get on the floor in a half-kneeling position, with one foot flat and the knee of the opposite leg on the ground behind you.
- Grasp the top of your back foot with both hands.
- Pull your heel toward your bottom while letting your hips sink forward into a deeper stretch.

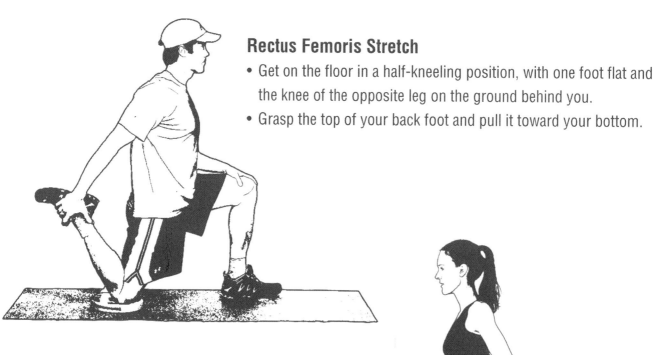

Rectus Femoris Stretch

- Get on the floor in a half-kneeling position, with one foot flat and the knee of the opposite leg on the ground behind you.
- Grasp the top of your back foot and pull it toward your bottom.

Lunge Stretch

- Take a large step forward into a lunge, with your front knee bent and your back leg straight.
- Allow the heel of your back leg to come off the ground.
- Drive your hips forward to feel a stretch in the thigh of your back leg.

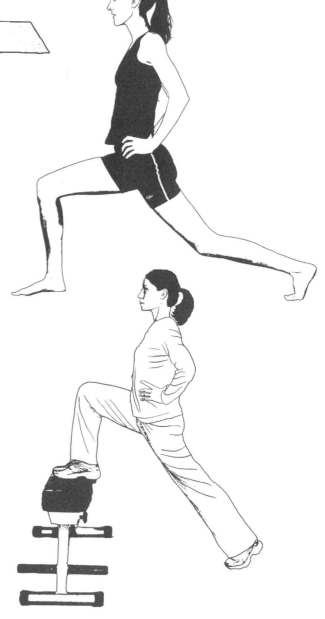

Leg Elevated Lunge

- Place your front foot on the top of a bench or box and extend your back leg.
- Drive your hips forward, sinking deeper into a lunge position.

Lunge Stretch with Sidebend

- Step forward into lunge, with your front knee bent and your back leg straight.
- Raise the arm on the same side as your back leg and perform a side bend toward the opposite side.

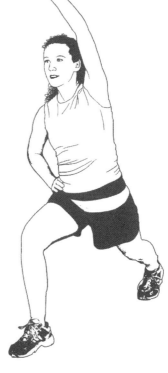

Deep Lunge Stretch

- Place one knee on the ground and step your other leg as far forward as it can go while still keeping your foot flat.
- Reach your hands to the floor and try to get your elbows to the ground.
- Let your hips sink downward.

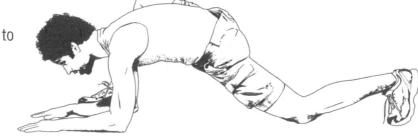

Pigeon Stretch

- Get on the ground with one leg extended behind you and your other leg tucked beneath you, with your outer thigh resting on the floor.
- Let your hips sink to the floor without rotating your body to the side.

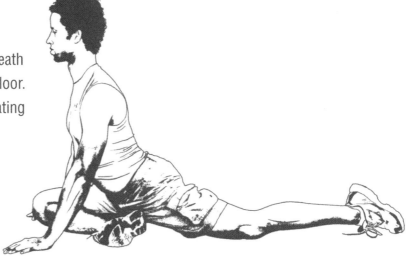

Advanced Pigeon

- Assume the same basic position as the Pigeon Stretch, but grasp the foot of your back leg.
- Pull your foot toward your bottom, stretching the knee behind you.

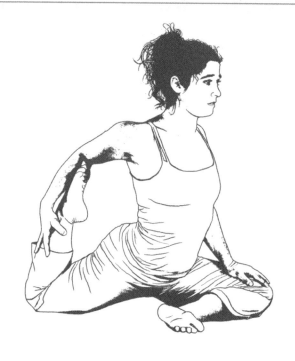

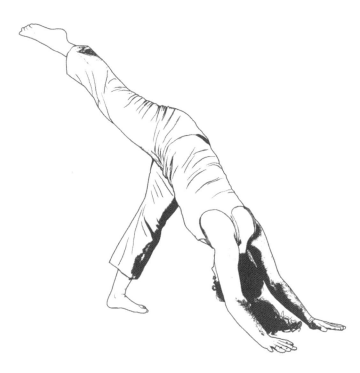

Overhead Leg Stretch

- From a standing position, place both hands on the floor.
- Position one leg a few feet behind you, keeping the foot flat.
- Lift your other leg to the ceiling as high as it will go.
- Drive your chest to the floor while lifting your hips higher.

Front Splits

- Get on the floor with one leg spread forward and the other one behind you.
- Ease your hips toward the ground.
- Use your hands on either side of your waist for support.

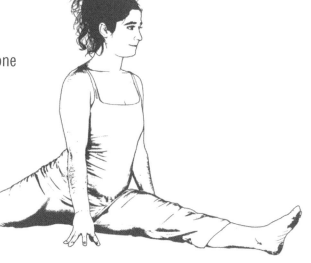

Kneeling TFL Stretch

- Assume a half-kneeling position next to a bench for support.
- Drive your hips forward while simultaneously leaning your trunk away from the bottom leg.
- *Variation:* Raise your outer arm overhead while completing the side-bend.

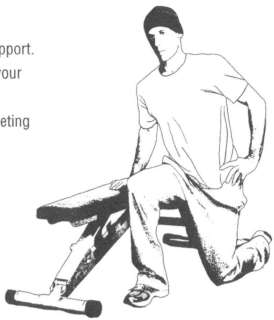

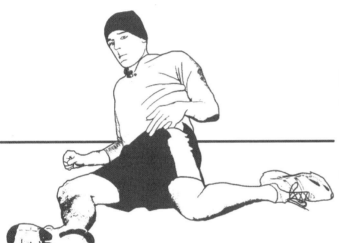

Reclined Hip Flexor Stretch

- Support yourself on the ground, resting on one elbow and with your legs split apart so the top leg is pulled backward.
- Pull the top leg farther backward to feel a stretch in the front of your thigh.

Supported Hip Flexor Stretch

- Support one leg behind you on a table, keeping your front foot on the floor.
- Press your hands into the table to lift your trunk.
- Drive your hips forward to stretch the thigh and groin of your back leg.

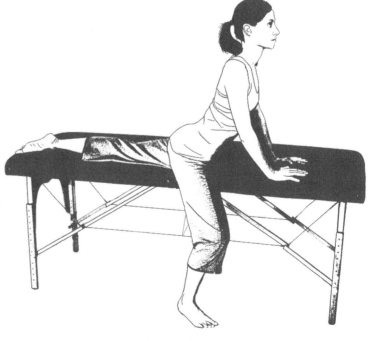

Table Hip Flexor Stretch

- Sit at the edge of a table and pull one knee to your chest while letting the other leg dangle off the edge.
- Let your trunk drop down to the table, keeping your knee pulled in to your chest.
- *Variation:* Have a partner help press your bottom leg lower, toward the floor.

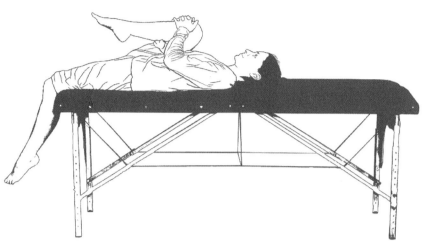

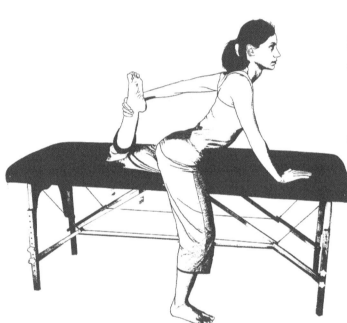

Supported Hip Flexor & Quad Stretch

- Get on a table in the same position as the Supported Hip Flexor Stretch, but grasp the foot of your back leg.
- Pull your foot to your bottom while keeping your thigh pressed into the table.

Groin Stretch

- Stand with your legs at least double shoulder-width apart.
- Lean toward one leg, bending the knee of that side, and rest your elbow on your thigh.
- Keep leaning away from your outstretched leg to stretch your inner thigh.

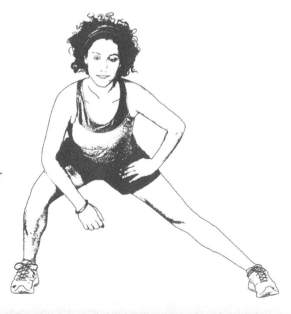

Groin & Hamstring Stretch

• Stand with your legs at least double shoulder-width apart.
• Bend one knee and squat toward that leg, keeping your other leg outstretched and resting on its heel.

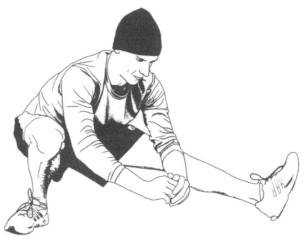

Side Splits

• Begin with your legs positioned greater than double shoulder-width apart.
• Let your hips sink toward the ground, spreading your feet wider apart.
• Reach your hands to the floor for support.

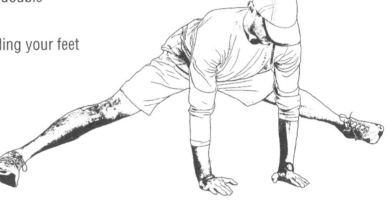

Wall Splits

• Lie on your back with your bottom pressed against a wall and your feet raised overhead.
• Allow your hips to relax and let your feet slide outward and apart against the wall.

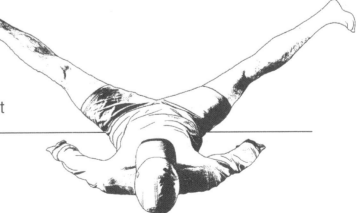

Butterfly Stretch

* Sit on the ground with your knees bent and your feet pulled into your groin.
* Grasp your ankles and use your elbows to press into your knees, spreading your thighs wider apart.
* Bend forward, bringing your chest closer to your feet.

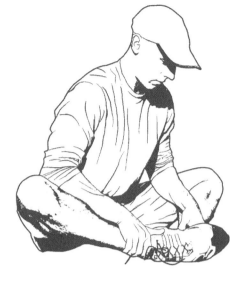

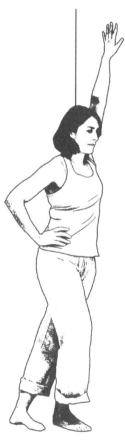
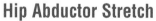
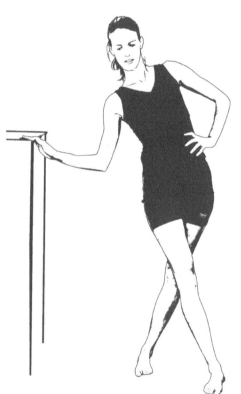

Hip Abductor Stretch

* Lean sideways with your closest arm resting overhead against a wall.
* Step your innermost leg behind your body, crossing the opposite ankle.
* Drop your hips toward the wall to feel a stretch of the innermost leg.

ITB Stretch

* Step one leg behind your body, crossing past the opposite leg.
* Drive your hips forward and toward the back leg.
* Use one hand to support your upper body on a wall or railing.

Crossed Leg ITB Stretch

- Lie on your back with your knees flexed.
- Cross one leg over the other and let your hips drop over to the side of the bottom leg.

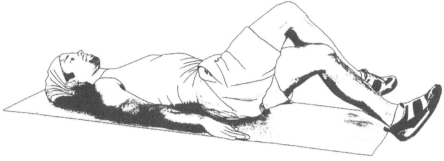

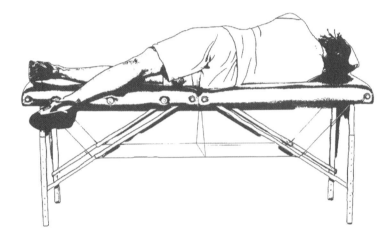

Side Lying ITB Stretch

- Lie on a table, resting on one side of your body.
- Let your top leg drop behind your body, off the table.
- Don't let your hips or trunk rotate backward.

Crossed Leg Forward Bend

- Cross one leg in front of the other, keeping both feet flat on the ground.
- Bend forward from your waist, reaching your hands to the floor.

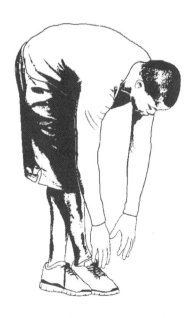

Hip Internal Rotation Stretch

- Lie on your back with your knees bent and both feet flat on the floor.
- Spread your thighs apart and let one knee drop inward toward the other.

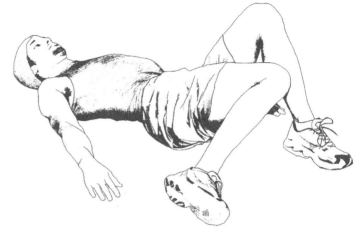

Cross-over Stretch

- Lie on your back with your arms spread wide.
- Lift one leg up and cross it over the opposite leg while keeping the knee straight.
- Keep your shoulders flat and try to reach the foot of your top leg to the floor.

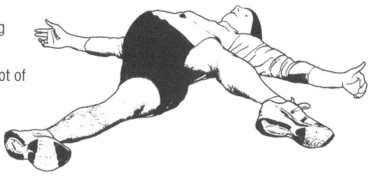

Glute / Piriformis Stretch

- Sit on the ground with your knees bent, resting backward on outstretched arms.
- Lift one leg and place your ankle on the opposite knee.
- Gently push your chest forward to drive your hips into a deeper stretch.

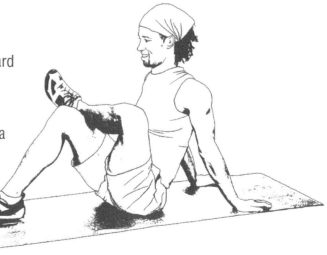

Dropped Hip Stretch

- Support your elbows on a bench, keeping your feet in front of your body and your hips elevated off the floor.
- Cross one ankle over the opposite knee.
- Slowly lower your hips to the floor for a deeper stretch.

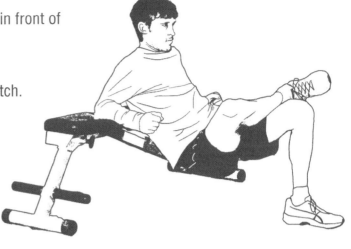

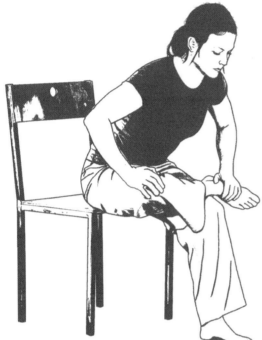

Seated Piriformis Stretch

- Sit on the floor with your legs extended in front of you.
- Grasp one knee and cross that leg over the other.
- Pull the knee to your chest to stretch your bottom.
- *Variation:* Grasp your ankle to help rotate your hip into a deeper stretch.

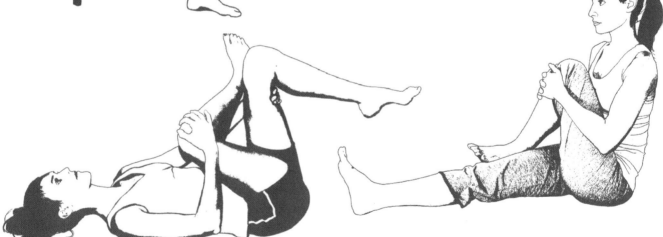

Piriformis Stretch

- Lie on your back with your knees bent and one ankle on the opposite thigh.
- Pull both legs up toward your chest to feel a stretch in your bottom.

Glute Stretch

- Sit on the floor with your legs extended in front of you.
- Grasp one knee and cross that leg over the other.
- Pull the knee to your chest, to stretch your bottom.
- *Variation:* Grasp your ankle to help rotate your hip into a deeper stretch.

Single Knee to Chest

- Lie on your back and use both hands to grasp one knee.
- Pull your knee toward your chest to feel a stretch in your hip and low back.

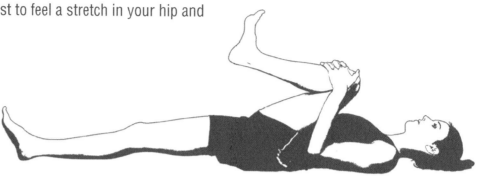

Double Knee to Chest

- Lie on your back and grasp both knees with your hands.
- Pull your knees toward your chest to feel a stretch in your hips and low back.

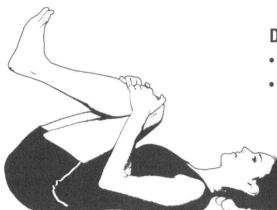

Forward Bend

- Stand with your feet spread shoulder-width apart.
- Hinge forward from your waist and reach your hands to the floor.
- Let your trunk dangle toward the ground.
- Make sure to breathe!

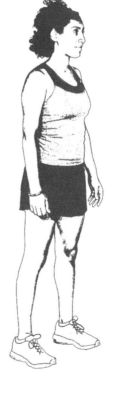
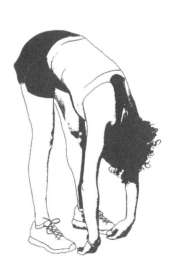

Squat Stretch

- Stand with your feet shoulder-width apart and toes pointed forward.
- Lower into a deep stretch, allowing your head to drop forward as well.
- Try to keep your heels on the floor, but let your hips open up to get as low as possible.

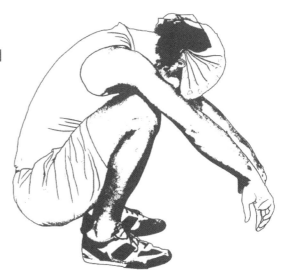

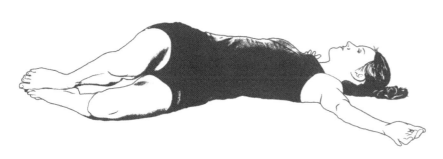

Lower Trunk Rotation

- Lie on your back with your knees bent and feet flat on the floor.
- Let your knees drop over to one side, rotating your lower trunk.
- Keep your upper back and shoulders flat against the ground.

Reclined Side Stretch

- Lie on your side with your bottom leg extended and your top leg bent.
- Place your hands on the ground near your chest and press downward to lift your trunk.

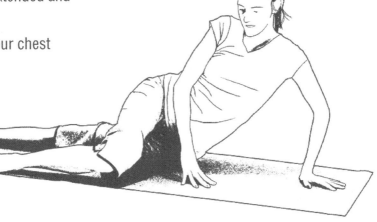

Standing Side Bend

- Stand with your feet spread slightly greater than shoulder-width apart.
- Perform a side bend by raising one hand toward the ceiling and dropping your other hand along the outside of your leg.

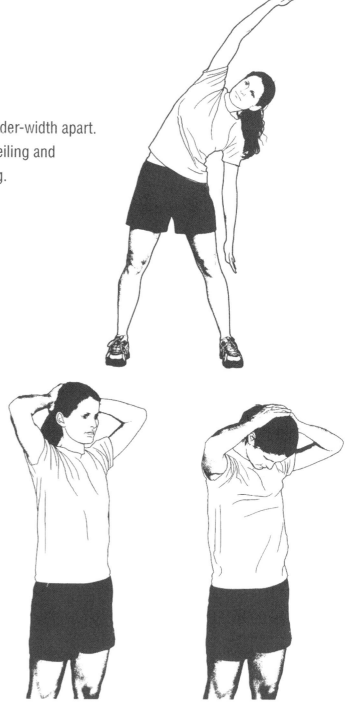

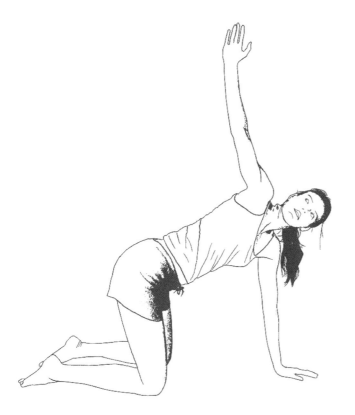

Kneeling Trunk Twist

- Get on all fours on the ground with your weight spread evenly between your hands and knees.
- Lift one arm from the floor, rotate your trunk to the side, and reach to the ceiling.
- *Variation:* Rather than lifting your arm upward, reach your hand between your opposite arm and leg.

Neck Flexion Stretch

- Interlace your fingers on the back of your head.
- Tuck your chin and gently pull your head forward, toward your chest.

Upper Trap Stretch

- Take one hand and grasp your head by the opposite temple.
- Pull your head directly to the side without letting it rotate.
- Hold the edge of a chair to prevent your opposite shoulder from rising.

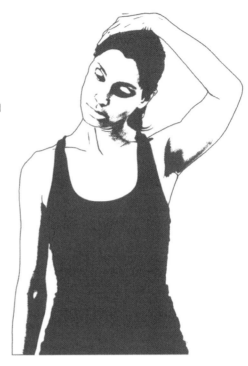

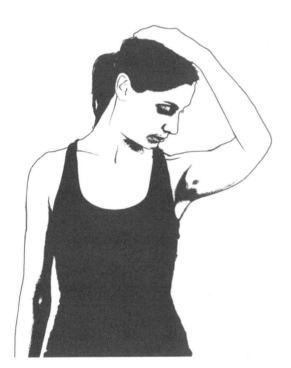

Levator Scapula Stretch

- Grasp the back of your head with one hand.
- Pull your face over to the side and downward, as if you were looking into your armpit.
- Keep your opposite shoulder from rising.

Levator Scap Stretch Variation

- Reach one hand over your shoulder and behind your back while grasping the back of your head with the other hand.
- Pull your head down and to the side, as if you were looking into your armpit.

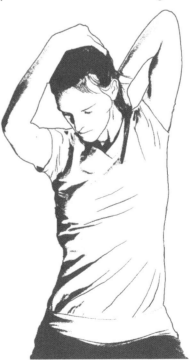

Shoulder & Neck Stretch

- Reach both arms behind your back and grasp one wrist with the opposite hand.
- Pull your shoulder downward and tilt your head in the opposite direction to stretch the side of your neck.

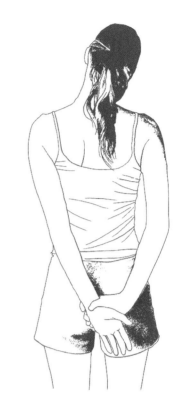

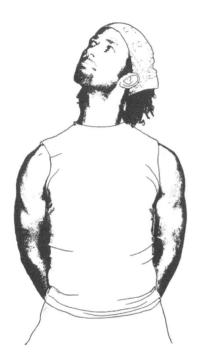

Scalene Stretch

- Secure your hands behind your back to keep your shoulders from rising.
- Lift your face up and to the side, so that you drop your head backward along a diagonal.
- You should feel a stretch on one side of the front of your neck.

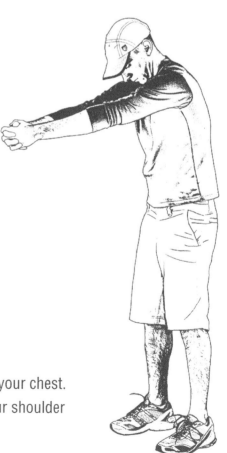

Upper Back Stretch

- Grasp your hands together and outstretch your arms in front of your chest.
- Drop your head and arch your back to feel a stretch between your shoulder blades.

Mid Back Stretch with Bench

- Place one knee on a bench and grasp the edge with your hand on the same side.
- Arch your back upward, pulling your shoulder away from your hand.
- *Make it harder*: Reach your hand through your body to grasp the opposite side of the bench.

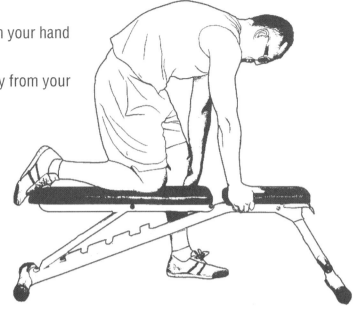

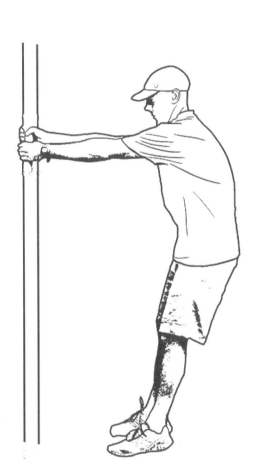

Mid Back Stretch with Bar

- Grasp a vertical bar or a doorframe with both hands.
- Arch your spine and drop your trunk backward to feel a stretch between your shoulder blades.

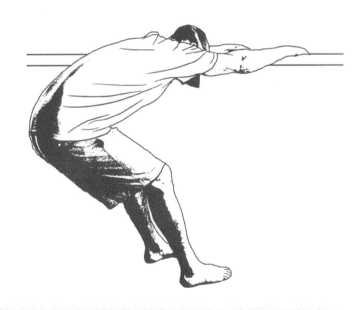

Shoulder & Back Stretch with Rail

- Grasp a horizontal bar with both hands spread shoulder-width apart.
- Sit backward and let your shoulders pull forward into an arm and mid-back stretch.

Lat Stretch

- Place both of your palms on a wall, spreading them shoulder-width apart.
- Walk your feet backward and drop your chest to feel a stretch beneath your shoulders.

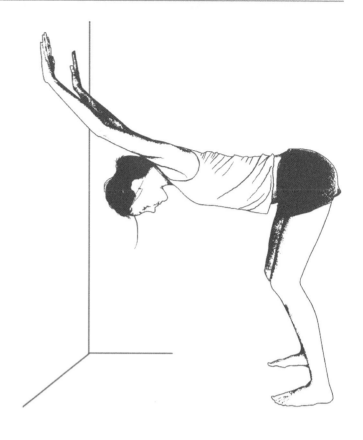

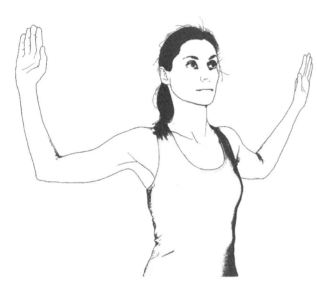

"W" Stretch

- Lift your elbows to the height of your shoulders, keeping your hands pointed to the ceiling.
- Pull your shoulder blades together to feel a stretch across your chest.
- *Variation:* Place your forearms on either side of a doorway and step your trunk through to stretch your chest.

Floor Shoulder & Chest Stretch

- Lie on your side with your bottom arm extended behind your body, palm-down.
- Gently rotate your trunk to the ceiling to feel a stretch in the front of your shoulder.

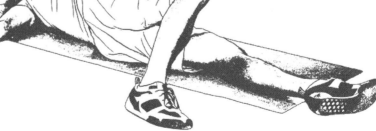

Macaco Stretch

- Get on the floor as if you were going to perform a Bridge-up.
- Extend one arm and press your hips to the ceiling.
- Reach toward the far wall with your opposite arm to feel a stretch along your side and shoulder.

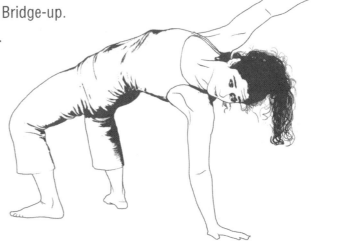

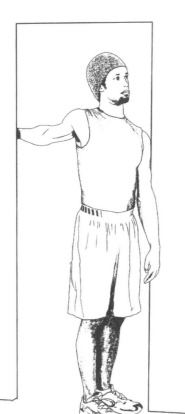

Doorway Shoulder & Chest Stretch

- Grab the edge of a doorframe (or vertical bar) with one arm and step forward, keeping the arm behind your body.
- Rotate your trunk away from your hand to stretch the front of your shoulder and chest.

Wall Shoulder & Chest Stretch

- Place one hand behind you against a wall, above the height of your shoulder.
- Rotate your trunk away from the wall to stretch your arm and chest.

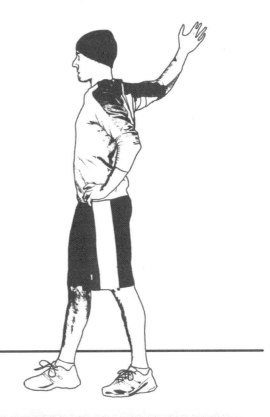

Reclined Shoulder Stretch

• Sit on the floor with both hands placed on the
  ground behind your back.
• Scoot your hips forward and drop your chest to feel
  a stretch of your shoulders.

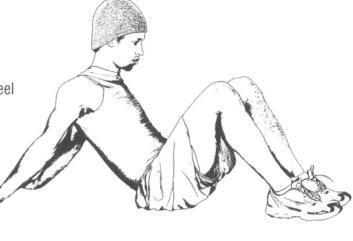

Pec Minor Stretch

• Sit at the edge of a bench with your hands placed
  near your hips.
• Allow your hips to come off the bench and drop
  your torso toward the floor.
• You should feel a stretch in your upper chest.

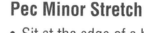

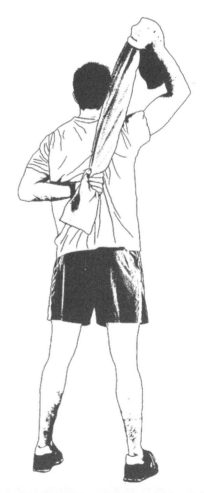

Towel Stretch

• Hold a towel behind your back, with one arm by your pelvis
  and the other by your head.
• Stretch your bottom shoulder by pulling the towel upward,
  easing your bottom hand up your spine.
• *Variation:* Stretch the upper shoulder by pulling the towel
  downward, easing your top hand between your shoulder
  blades.

Tricep Stretch

- Raise both arms above your head and grasp the elbow of one arm with your opposite hand.
- Flex your elbow as far as it will go and pull the arm over to the opposite side for a deeper stretch.

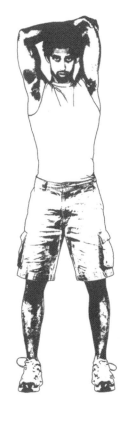

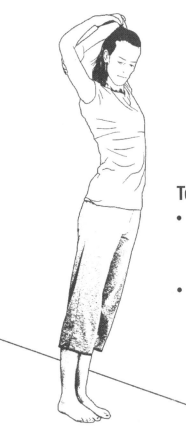

Teres Major Stretch

- Lean into a wall with one arm raised overhead, resting against your outer shoulder.
- Use your other arm to help pull the elbow farther to the side to feel a stretch beneath your armpit.

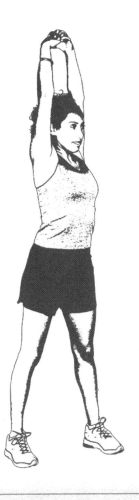

Overhead Shoulder Stretch

- Raise both arms overhead and interlace your fingers.
- Press your hands to the ceiling while pulling your arms backward and driving your chest forward.

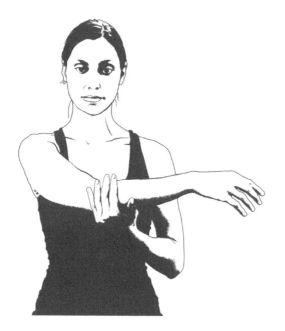

Posterior Shoulder Stretch

- Use one hand to grasp the elbow of your opposite arm.
- Pull the arm across your body to feel a stretch on the back of your shoulder.
- *Variation:* Let your shoulder blade glide forward to stretch your mid-back.

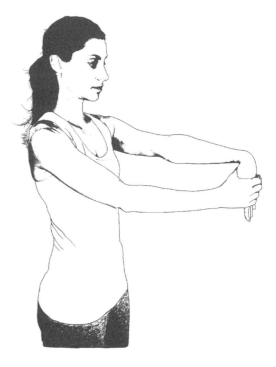

Wrist Flexion Stretch

- Grasp the back of one hand with the opposite hand and extend both arms forward from your body.
- Pull your fingers downward while keeping your elbows straight to feel a stretch on the top of your forearm.

Wrist Extension Stretch

- Grasp your palm and the fingers of one hand with your opposite hand and extend your elbows.
- Pull your hand backward while keeping your arms straight to feel a stretch in your forearm.

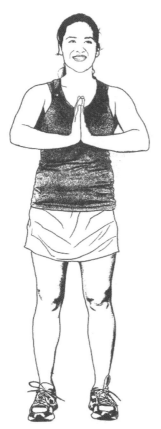

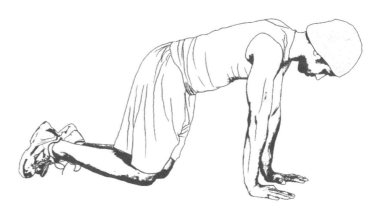

Kneeling Wrist Extension

- Kneel on the ground and place your palms flat with the fingers pointed forward.
- Gently drive your body forward, bringing your shoulders over your wrists.

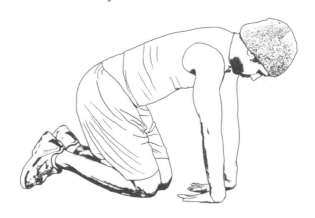

Prayer Stretch

- Press the palms of both hands together and in front of your chest.
- Apply pressure while driving your hands down and bringing your elbows upward.
- *Variation:* Reverse the stretch by pressing the back of your hands together, and then lifting your hands and dropping your elbows.

Kneeling Wrist Flexion

- Kneel on the ground and place the back of your hands on the ground, with your fingers pointed toward your knees.
- Carefully sit your weight backward, stretching your wrists into deeper flexion.

Wrist Supination Stretch

- Grasp one hand below your thumb at your wrist and apply pressure on the back of the hand to rotate your pinky inward toward your face.
- Straighten your arm to take the stretch deeper.
- *Variation:* Reverse your hand placement to rotate your palm away from your face, into pronation.

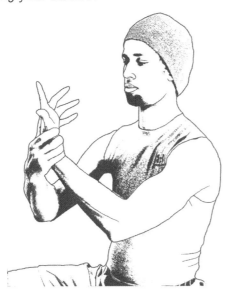

Chapter 14

"Once you understand the main principles of how to cook up a killer workout, you'll never feel bored in your fitness pursuits."

Cooking it up

AKA: How to create killer workouts

You have in your hands an enormous collection of exercises. Do yourself a favor, and recall the basic premise of this encyclopedia: *The broader array of movement skills that you train, the better athlete you will be.* Think of the 700+ movements as the ingredients from which you can cook up an infinite variety of workouts. By combining the different skills into effective workouts, you can take your physical ability and athletic prowess to new heights.

Although *Mad Skills* is not a fitness cookbook, providing the workout ingredients for specific recipes, we will still explore a few concepts of workout design. Once you understand the main principles of how to cook up a killer workout, you'll never feel bored in your fitness pursuits.

General Athleticism versus Sport Specificity

Quick reminder: If you want to become a better all-around athlete, someone who can easily flip-flop between a trail run, a game of ultimate, or an impromptu wrestling match, then you are wise to work on your general athleticism. The types of workouts that will be described below are those types of workouts. They are designed to get you ready for all of life's challenges.

If, on the other hand, you are seeking a way to get better at just one specific sport or skill set, then you need a different, more tailored approach. A track and field competitor trying to win gold in the high jump would likely be wasting her time goofing around on gymnastics rings. For the average Joe or Jane it is wise to pursue a broader approach to fitness. And, yet, for an athlete in competitive mode, specificity is ideal.

Main Guidelines for Workout Design

Warm-up

It is crucial that you prepare your body prior to any intense physical effort. If you don't, you will get hurt. Period.

Pick one or two of the warm-up activities from the first chapter and perform them for at least 5 to 10 minutes before starting the bulk of your workout. Your heart rate and breathing rate should increase. A light sweat should form. Your joints should be limbered up. And your muscles should be neurologically stimulated—ready for action.

Strive for balance

When you choose exercises for your workouts, you should pay equal attention to your upper body, lower body, and core/trunk. It goes without saying that you also need to strive for symmetry from the left side to the right side. Likewise, you want to focus equal efforts on both sides of a joint —some muscles push a limb away from you, while others pull it toward you. If you neglect to take a balanced approach to what muscles you use, deficiencies will arise and your performance will decline.

Now, performing an effective workout that hits every muscle group in equal parts would take forever. That's not what is being advocated. Instead, try to be balanced in what muscles you use over a series of workouts. Over the course of a week or two, you should be able to cycle through enough movement variety to be truly comprehensive.

- For example, a workout of pull-ups, lunges, and hollow rocking meets the basic criteria for a single session. But, if that were all you did for a week straight, then you would have neglected your chest, triceps, calves, hamstrings, and back extensors.

- Similarly, push-ups, shoulder presses, and bent-over rows done together don't make for a balanced workout. But, if you did squats, stiff-leg deadlifts, and reverse hyperextensions on the following day, you would be on the right path overall.

Compound movements

The main lifts in each workout should be compound, multi-joint movements. Moving your body through space efficiently depends on the coordinated action of multiple body parts. If your workouts don't incorporate this type of movement, you'll fail to make appreciable gains in performance.

Lower body compound skills:

- Squats
- Deadlifts
- Step-ups
- Lunges
- Jumping

Upper body compound skills:

- Pull-ups (and muscle-ups)
- Push-ups
- Chest and shoulder presses
- Rowing variations (bent-over or with body-weight on rings or bar)
- Dips

Whole body compound skills:

- Clean + clean and press
- Overhead squat, lunge, get-up
- Thruster and push-press
- Snatch
- Swing
- Turkish get-up
- Burpee

Make it a habit to include at least one or two of the movements listed above, in each workout.

Exercise variety

One goal of your workout design is that you should cycle through at least 1/3 of the different exercises in this encyclopedia at least once a year. Compound movements should always be the foundation of how you develop strength, yet periodically sprinkling in isolation exercises or subtle variations to foot/hand placement helps prepare your body for a mix of physical demands. Comb through each chapter and try to add one or two unique skill per workout.

Use these questions to steer your movement selection:

- **Is there variety in the modalities that you choose?** Over the course of many workouts, try to use everything in your arsenal. Use a pull-up bar, dumbbells, medicine balls, parallettes, rings, kettlebells, barbells, and even a sandbag.

- **What is the mix of static versus dynamic strength?** Isometric skills like planks and V-sits, or gymnastic holds like planches and levers, are a crucial means to develop whole body strength. Disregard them at your own peril.

- **Are you including explosive movements?** Whether you throw a medicine ball, do box jumps, or work on clapping push-ups, some component of your workout structure should include explosive or plyometric muscle action.

- **Can you design a workout by limiting yourself to just one tool?** Limiting yourself to just one piece of equipment is a fun way to create variety in your workouts. For instance, what are three different movements you could do with a park bench? This is a skill that comes in handy when you're on vacation and want to do a quick workout!

- **Do you vary from single limb to dual limb lifts and movements?** In real life, we don't always have the opportunity to lift or move with both limbs in unison. Aside from mimicking real-life movement, unilateral skills help you develop stability and core strength.

The list of 10 General Physical Skills revered by CrossFit athletes and attributed to Jim Crawley and Bruce Evans is a great tool to help steer your exercise selection. Incorporate enough movement variety that you touch upon all of these skills, and you are sure to improve your fitness and become a more complete athlete.

1. Endurance	6. Speed
2. Stamina	7. Coordination
3. Strength	8. Agility
4. Flexibility	9. Balance
5. Power	10. Accuracy

Circuit structure

At the most basic level, your workouts should center on a circuit of a few different exercises, somewhere between 3 and 5 different skills. Ideally, they will include a mix of upper body, lower body, and core/trunk movements. You will always warm-up for a few minutes prior to the circuit, and then it is up to you how you wish to cool down or recover.

Here is how to choose what exercises go in the circuit:

- **Main exercises:** Pick 1 or 2 compound movements as the meat and potatoes of your workout. These are the exercises where you will be challenging the greatest number of muscle groups, and consequently where you will fatigue yourself the greatest. If you want to do two compound movements, split them between your upper and lower body.

- **Supplemental exercises:** Pick another 2 to 3 exercises to supplement the muscle action of your main lifts. These exercises are where you can get creative— select from isometric skills, plyometric movements, single limb drills, or isolated joint action. They can mimic the muscle actions of the main exercises, but should be of a much lesser difficulty. Better yet, choose exercises that target completely different muscles from the main lifts.

As a general rule, if you want to do just a very basic circuit training workout, choose a mix of exercises and perform them for enough sets that you *end up doing between 9 and 16 sets.* On the low end, 3 exercises rotated through 3 times would give you a nice and short circuit. On the upper end, 4 different exercises rotated 4 times through would give you a longer and more strenuous workout. There are many reasons why you might want to choose a different arrangement, but as a basic rule, the 9–16 set organization is very helpful.

- **Set combos to try** (# of exercises in the circuit x # of rotations through the circuit): 3 x 3, 3 x 4, 3 x 5, 4 x 3, 4 x 4, 5 x 3

- **Timed intervals:** Instead of doing a predetermined number of reps for each station of a circuit, try doing one or all stations as a timed interval. For instance, do hollow rocks for 60 seconds, pull-ups for 30 seconds, and split jumps for 45 seconds.

> If you would like a visual resource for how to organize different movements into a basic circuit training workout, see the website StrengthMob.com.

Vary your emphasis

Just as if you stuck with only one set of movements in each workout, if you did only one type of circuit over the course of many weeks, things would get old fast. Plus, by emphasizing different aspects of your workout design, you condition your body to prepare for a variety of different demands.

Experiment with placing emphasis on each of these aspects:

- **For time ("as fast as possible")**: After you do your warm-up, hustle to get through the prescribed sets and repetitions of each exercise, as fast as you can. Take out your stopwatch and challenge yourself to crank through the workout in blazing speed.

- **For rounds (AMRAP—"as many rounds as possible")**: Set a time limit, say 10 minutes, and then try to crank through as many rounds of the circuit as you can. If you were doing a circuit with 4 exercises, you would try to cycle through the 4 movements as many times as possible during the time limit, while performing the designated number of reps.

- **For quality**: Designate the number of repetitions for each skill that you want to perform, and then execute each movement with perfect form. Repetitions in which you break form do not count to the total number. This is a great workout structure for body-weight skills. An example workout would be to collect 30 handstand push-ups, 20 muscle-ups, and 3 minutes of L-sit on the rings.

- **For weight**: In this workout, you would push yourself to lift your maximal amount of weight on each exercise. If you were doing squats and kettlebell shoulder presses, you would try to use the heaviest weight that you could for the prescribed number of repetitions.

- **For reps**: Do a workout where the point is just to get through a ridiculous number of repetitions of each exercise. Something like 300 crunches, 200 body-weight squats, and 50 pull-ups would be a good example.

Go hard!

No matter how beautiful your workout design, if you don't push yourself to go hard during it, you won't make gains in your performance. To see improvements in strength and power you must absolutely challenge yourself. Anything less than full effort during a workout is a waste of time.

So, how "hard" is hard?

In terms of weight lifting, this means that you are moving enough weight that you are fatigued and near failure at the end of the prescribed number of reps. Go hard enough that if you tried to do an extra one or two reps you would lose form, causing a deterioration of your technique. Injuries occur when form breaks down, so you should obviously stop before that point.

For the purpose of power development, something that is critical for all athletes, you want to lift enough weight that you reach fatigue at a range between 8 to 12 reps. If you want to make bigger gains in pure strength and muscle mass, lower that number down (and add weight) so that you reach fatigue at 3 to 6 reps. Beware: The heavier weight takes a greater toll on your body, and you will potentially be sore for days!

The smart use of recovery periods and additional mobility training takes on greater importance when you begin to lift heavier and heavier weights.

When you aim to build strength with body-weight skills, a different approach is needed—you can't just keep adding weight plates. As skills become too easy, meaning you can crank out over a dozen reps without fatigue, you generally need to start loading your muscles with a greater and greater proportion of your body's mass. A simple example is to move from incline (chest-elevated) push-ups, to regular push-ups, and then decline (feet-elevated) push-ups. After that, you could do jackknife push-ups, and eventually handstand push-ups.

Adding a weight vest is generally a good next phase for when you feel you have maxed out with basic body-weight skills. It's either that or you can start to explore the super advanced movements used by competitive gymnasts, like the iron cross on the rings.

If you are interested in learning more about workout programming for strength gains, check out the recommended reading at the end of this chapter. So much has already been written about the art and science of weight lifting and strength development, that it would be a waste of paper to explore it any more in this exercise encyclopedia.

Do it together

A special alchemy occurs when people get together to exercise as a community. When you have a training partner or a group of friends to exercise with, it's inevitable that you'll push yourself harder than if you were doing it alone. With your buddies around you, you're less likely to skimp on weight, reps, or simply quit early. The extra motivation yields a more effective workout overall.

Added benefits of working out in a group include the following:

- **Stress relief:** People are social animals. When we exercise as a tribe, we can decompress from the stresses of work life.

- **Accountability:** An established workout schedule is an excellent tool to keep you on track with your fitness. It's a lot harder to bail on a workout when you know that you have people counting on you to show up.

- **Partner skills:** Having just one extra person present during your workout opens up a whole new world of movement possibilities. Medicine ball tosses and fireman carries can't be done alone!

- **Spotting:** When you challenge yourself with a heavy weight or a new movement skill, it's often a good idea to have a second person "spot" you for safety. Aside from being there to prevent injury, a spotter can also call out positional flaws to help you improve your technique.

Rest and Recovery

Just as the warm-up is a crucial pre-workout activity, so is adequate rest and recovery after the workout ends. On the micro level, giving the main muscle groups used in a workout a day off before challenging them again, with significant effort, is always wise. On the macro level, after going hard in your training for many weeks (or months) on end, it's smart to give yourself a rest week. If you don't account for adequate rest, your nervous and hormonal systems will eventually become over-taxed, leading to a deterioration of your skills.

The term "overtraining" is used to describe the state when you have been going hard for too long, and your physical performance actually begins to decline. As someone who loves to move, you must be careful to avoid overtraining, as it will prevent you from moving well. Avoid it at all costs.

In between your workouts, select stretches and yoga postures from chapters 12 and 13 to help maintain your flexibility, posture, and general alignment. Failure to keep your body limber will counteract all of the good work you have been doing to build strength and power. Also, mobility work with bands, balls, and foam rollers is something you should explore further.

Sleep and nutrition are the final pieces to the rest and recovery puzzle. Make sure to let your body completely recuperate with sufficient sleep and fuel it with high quality meals. If you refill your energy tank with junk food and crummy sleep, you're going to get poor performance out of your body.

Forget everything, and just move!

It is natural to feel overwhelmed when considering all of the variables that can go into workout structure and the pursuit of human performance. Likewise, it is easy to fall into the trap of just exercising for the sake of exercise. Yet, who cares if you create killer workouts and go hard all the time, but you aren't having fun?

If the past few pages and hundreds of different exercises have your head spinning, worry not. Forget it all if you want.

Movement is the answer.

You're holding the largest illustrated exercise encyclopedia the world has ever seen, but it barely skims the surface of the infinite variety of ways that humans can move. Let the hundreds of exercises in here be the jumping off point for your own discoveries of what your body can accomplish. By mixing things up and tying different exercises together, you'll undoubtedly come up with hundreds of more movements that could be in future editions of *Mad Skills*.

Above all, remember the reason why you choose to exercise in the first place: It is to hone your body into a more capable vehicle for the pursuit of whatever sports or movement-skills that bring you joy. A weak and inflexible body cannot compete with the performance of a strong and limber one. Choose to craft your body into the finest performance vehicle that it can become.

When you're at a loss for what to do next with your fitness or you've grown stagnant with working out, JUST GO PLAY. Explore new ways to move your body. Try to add an original movement to your growing skill-set. Come up with physical challenges that test the limits of how you can move.

> *Your journey ends when your chest fails to rise with new breath.*
>
> *Movement is an inherent feature of life; its absence is death.*
>
> *Never stop moving.*

Recommended reading:

- *Athletic Body in Balance: Optimal Movement Skills and Conditioning for Performance*, by Gray Cook.

- *Becoming a Supple Leopard: The Ultimate Guide to Resolving Pain, Preventing Injury, and Optimizing Athletic Performance*, by Kelly Starrett and Glen Cordoza.

- *Exuberant Animal: The Power of Health, Play and Joyful Movement*, by Frank Forencich

- *Kettlebell Rx: The Complete Guide for Athletes and Coaches*, by Jeff Martone.

- *Olympic Weightlifting: A Complete Guide for Athletes and Coaches*, by Greg Everett.

- *Overcoming Gravity: A Systematic Approach to Gymnastics and Bodyweight Strength*, by Steven Low and Valentin Uzunov.

- *Power, Speed, Endurance: A Skill-based Approach to Endurance Training*, by Brian MacKenzie and Glen Cordoza.

- *Practical Programming for Strength Training*, by Mark Rippetoe and Lon Kilgore.

- *The 4-Hour Body: An Uncommon Guide to Rapid Fat-loss, Incredible Sex, and Becoming Superhuman*, by Timothy Ferris.

- *Why We Run: A Natural History*, by Bernd Heinrich.

Acknowledgements

First and foremost, I must thank my wonderful family, including my parents, Ed and Mary, my sister, Laura, and my wife, Lorraine. Any accomplishments on my account, including this book, are due to your ceaseless support. You have always had faith in my endeavors and I owe it all to you.

To the people who helped make this project come together, including Diego Diaz, Miguel Aldana, Kara Aldana, Kristin Russ, Martin Schoeneborn, and all of the models: It's been a pleasure working with you, and thanks for putting up with me!

I need to give a big shout out to the entire Beyond the Clinic crew, especially Aaron Saari and Bryan Pasternak. My Finn and Master Pasters, you have both taught me so much about exercise and life. I'm grateful to have you on my team!

Sensei Patrick Murphy, you had an enormous impact on the development of my discipline and athletic ability. My elementary school-aged self bows to you.

Ramman Turner, thanks for pushing me and sharing your knowledge.

Erik Newgard, your building skills helped BPM Rx, Inc. get off the ground in more ways than one. You are an awesome friend.

To my Portland friends, including everyone from Grupo de Capoeira Regional do Brasil and the Strength Mob: You brighten life in the Pacific Northwest—thanks for holding the rain at bay.

For all of the friends who I've made over the different phases of this life, although we may be apart now, you are all still in my heart.

Finally, to all of my past, present, and future training partners: Whether we spar, practice aerials, or shred on a board, thanks for moving with me.

Here is to a life of movement and play!

Massive thanks to all the crowd-funding donors!

Supporter

Dylan Akinrele
Miguel Aldana
Beth Anderson
Oleg Baranovsky
Jeff Barton
Becky Berkan
Michael Bernstein
Todd Bertges
Johann, Chris & Isaac Bibro
Andrew Binsack
Michael J. Bishop, DPT
Leanne Boggs
Ethan Breckenridge
Catriona Buhayar
Ionut Callini
Daniel Carrasco
Willis Chinn
William J. Clarke
John Conklin II
Alex Conrad
Alicia Crockett
Michael Darlington-West
Paul "Diddy" Darnell
Dayna Dawson
Ann Dempsey
Brandon Diaz Pineda
Molly Dolezalek
Winston Dunn
Daniel Durham
Rob Elrod
Alli Fairbanks
Derek Fenwick
Dr. Casey Frieder
Sandra Friedman & Family
Viktor "The Beast" Foote
Ryan Ford
Greg Forehand
Tomas Galicia
Chris Garay

Al Gensitskiy
Roe Goodman
Mary Gramling
Benjamin B. Grandy
Pedro Guerra &
WheelHouse Fitness
Eli & Rayna Green
Roger Gremminger
Kasem Nithipatikom
Markus Heinesen
Jared Hinkley
Mark Hoffman
Tony Hope
Elliot Hulse & Strength Camp
Vince Kingston
Anna Long
Michele Limpens
Bill Madill
Sue Malone
Brent McCaskill
Jessica Miller
Lindsey Mockel
Travis Moe &
Shannon Sinsheimer, ND
Jeremiah Moore
Alfredo V. Moreno
Tom Mountjoy
Anne Moreau
Kirk Newgard
Thomas O'Donnell
Tasha Parman, DPT
Jamie & Senna Pinney
Frank Pederson
Ryan Pennington
Iñaky Pérez González
Nathan Pierce
Mike Phillips
Jutta Reichardt
Stephen Ristau
Mathew Roark
Jonathan Roberts

J. Nicholas Sarris
Travis Scott
Carson Sloan
Paul Smith
Dean Stegeman
Barbara Stephenson
Emily Tarter
Andrew & Sara Thompson
Jason Tippets
Joseph Trader, M.D.
Ramman Turner & Primordial Playground
Rich Urmy Jr.
Kjell van Zoen
Morgan Weisz
Per Widén
Adam Woodford
Eric Wong & First Cut Fitness

Benefactor

Rubyna Brenden
Bennette Burks
Deb & Mike Gaffney
Patrick Hentges
Christina Howell
Mark Kats
Demian Knight
Eric Luer
Ed Musholt
Laura Musholt
Mary Musholt
Erik Newgard & Sara Mohkami
Sasha Rotecki

Patron

Matt Antis
Bryan Pasternak
Aaron Saari

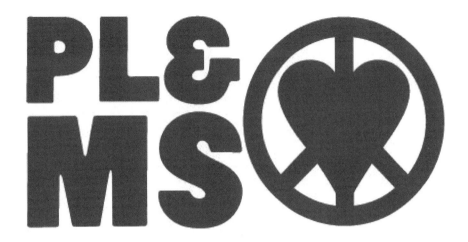

The world always needs more Peace, Love and Mad Skills.

If you would like access to additional content, including a hidden chapter and workout examples, all you have to do is help share *Mad Skills* with your friends!

Perform the actions below to access the additional content:

1. Share a link to the book with your Facebook friends.
    REWARD: Chapter 15 - Prehab Skills
2. Share a link to the book with your Twitter followers.
    REWARD: 10 body-weight workouts
3. Write an Amazon review of the Mad Skills Exercise Encyclopedia.
    REWARD:15 free-weight and kettlebell workouts
4. Do a YouTube review of the book.
    REWARD: Strength Mob sticker pack
5. Write a review of the book on your personal blog.
    REWARD: 30 minute Skype consult with the author
6. Tag an exercise picture/video of yourself on Instagram, Twitter, or Vine with hashtag #madskillsbook.
    REWARD: Enter a contest to win a Strength Mob T-shirt.

You can do one or all of the above actions—it's your call. Anything is helpful!

Chapter 15 and the 2 workout packs will be provided as digital downloads (PDF).

For details visit:
www.MadSkillsBook.com

Are you someone who prescribes exercise for a living?

Would you like to use the images in *Mad Skills* with your clients?

Use coupon code: "MadSkills" to receive 50% off the monthly subscription cost to:

www.BPMRx.com

Join the thousands of other coaches, personal trainers, and physical therapists, who are already using it!

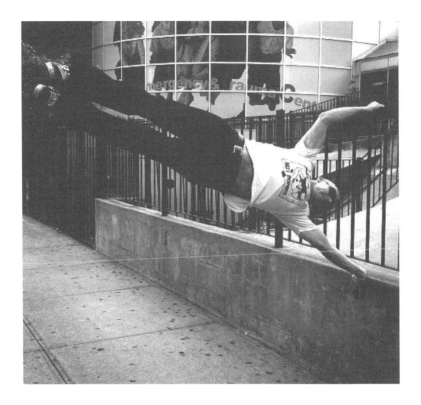

Ben Musholt is a licensed physical therapist and APEX Movement certified Parkour and Freerunning coach in Portland, Oregon. He is a co-founder of the *Beyond the Clinic* rehabilitation practice, and also runs *BPM Rx, Inc.* His writing has been featured on the *Men's Fitness* and *Breaking Muscle* websites. He also blogs at ParkourConditioning.com and posts workouts to StrengthMob.com.

His goal is to do 3 fun physical activities each day. Try to keep up!

Facebook: MadSkillsBook

Twitter: BPMRx

YouTube: BPMRx